My First Year as a Doctor

MY FIRST YEAR AS A DOCTOR

REAL-WORLD STORIES
FROM
AMERICA'S M.D.'s

Edited By

MELISSA RAMSDELL

WALKER AND COMPANY
NEW YORK

First published in the United States of America in 1994 by Walker Publishing Company, Inc.

Published simultaneously in Canada by Thomas Allen & Son Canada, Limited, Markham, Ontario

Library of Congress Cataloging-in-Publication Data
My first year as a doctor: real-world stories from America's M.D.'s
edited by Melissa Ramsdell.
p.   cm.
Includes index.
ISBN 0-8027-1290-8 (cloth).—ISBN 0-8027-7418-0 (pbk.)
I. Physicians—United States.   2. Medicine—Anecdotes.
I. Ramsdell, Melissa.
[DNLM: I. Physicians—United States—personal narratives.   WZ 112
M995   1994]
R690.M94   1994
610.69'52'0973—dc20
DNLM/DLC
for Library of Congress   94-4990
CIP

Book design by Glen M. Edelstein

Printed in the United States of America

2   4   6   8   10   9   7   5   3   I

Contents

Foreword

How could I read this delightful book without pausing to reflect on my own first year in medical practice? The place was Lower Greasewood, a settlement on the Navajo reservation in northeastern Arizona. The time was 1972. The characters were much, much younger.

I was the only physician at an Indian Health Service facility that served a large boarding school for Navajo children and thousands of people scattered over hundreds of square miles of arid steppe and high plateau. My wife and I lived with our two young children in a trailer nestled in a grove of cottonwoods about 200 yards from the clinic. I'd frequently see seventy to eighty patients in a day, some of whom were very sick, some of whom just rode into town to socialize a few hours at the trading post and pick up a new bottle of "big red pills" for their aches and pains. There were days I'd walk home lightly in the evening with my heart singing, "This is the life for me!" There were also days on which I'd walk home feeling incompetent, overworked, and overwhelmed. I remember weekends when my family and I would drive three hours to Flagstaff just to camp out in a cheap motel. We'd watch TV (those were the days before satellite dishes brought television to places like Lower Greasewood), cook our meals on the Coleman stove, and gratefully sleep without the threat of midnight knocks at our door—mothers with sick kids, drunks beaten up on the way home.

During that year at Lower Greasewood I learned what it means to be a physician—not in terms of scientific knowledge or abstract virtue, but in the day-to-day events that make up a life story. I had entered a profession, not simply taken a job. Somewhere in the great human story of healing I had taken my place as an uncertain and insignificant character. My story was not entirely my own anymore: I had obligations to patients, to the Navajo community, and to the medical profession itself. Of course, these realizations didn't help quench my anger very much when awakened in the middle of the night by a patient's staccato knock.

That was more than twenty years ago. I think it was easier then for young physicians to understand that stories are the core of medical practice—stories of sickness and suffering, traditions of healing, the day-to-day narratives of physicians trying to make their way in a difficult profession. Nowadays young people arriving at medical school have to overcome two powerful cultural myths before they can accept the "story-ness" of medicine. The first myth is that medicine is a commodity and physicians are its salespeople. We encounter this metaphor daily in insidious phrases like, "health care consumers" and "providers." Of course, medical practice was a business in 1972, just as it had been in the days of Hippocrates, Sydenham, and Osler. But in the past twenty years, the financial rewards and administrative rigmarole of medical practice have grown so greatly that the general public—and perhaps some aspiring medical trainees as well—is confused about what comes first: the personal commitment to healing or the bottom line.

The second myth is that medical practice is nothing but applied science and therefore just a matter of pushing the right button or prescribing the right drug. Balderdash! Unfortunately, our profession has become a victim of its own successes. Scientific and technological developments have had such a profound effect on medicine that we tend to forget the "heart" of our endeavor: alleviating the suffering of illness and caring for sick people. Machines simply can't do the job.

It is hoped that young physicians learn the limits of these myths as they immerse themselves in patients' stories. They learn thousands of facts, hundreds of skills, but most important they learn the values that motivate and sustain medical practice. These values—compassion, benevolence, respect, courage, honesty, humility—are not found in textbooks. They are learned in ordinary, day-to-day interactions with patients, peers, and teachers. The physician's identity as a healer—which is to say, his or her personal story—develops gradually over a period of years, both before and after medical school graduation. The M.D. degree may christen one a "doctor," but it is only a step along the way of professional development.

My First Year as a Doctor is an inspiring book because it illustrates the story of medicine and its values as embodied in the experience of wonderfully different people. At one level, the book gives us a practical assessment of what's to be expected "out there" for physicians starting practice, a guide to the ups and downs of the first year as experienced by a varied group of generalists and specialists. The expected and unexpected, the personal and political, the handy tip and the wise caution all emerge from these interesting tales.

At another level, however, *My First Year as a Doctor* is a book of stories about healing and professional values. And how fascinating are the tales these doctors tell! David Preston, newly arrived in a small town in Maine, experiences the thrill of making a correct diagnosis and seeing his grateful patient restored to health. For Edward Dow, an oncologist, there is no uncertainty about his patient's diagnosis or prognosis. The woman is dying of Hodgkin's disease. Dow's accomplishment is quite different from Preston's: helping family members through the trauma of deciding about continued life support for their comatose loved one. In California, David Simenson learns to understand his patients' narratives by reaching across cultural barriers, while Brenda Merritt learns to find a "person" deserving of respect in each of her patients at a South Bronx emergency room. Debra Williams, running a clinical studies program in a pharmaceutical company, demonstrates compassion by making an experimental AIDS drug available to a suffering child, while Steve Vogelsang learns humility from a sixty-eight-year-old diabetic woman who lives in a one-room shack in the mountains of eastern Kentucky.

As a medical educator, I often wonder what's really happening out there in the real world. Are our young physicians moving beyond the popular myths that medicine is simply a business or a technical skill? Are our graduates internalizing the traditional values of medicine? Are their stories as interesting and edifying as I had hoped they would be? Judging from *My First Year as a Doctor*, the answers are all positive. As we move into a difficult era of health care reform, the future of medicine has many uncertainties, but one thing is clear from this book: Our new practitioners are right on target. Bravo! Encore!

> —John L. Coulehan, M.D.,
> School of Medicine,
> State University of New York,
> Stony Brook

Acknowledgments

This book would not have been possible without the physicians who took time away from their hectic work schedules and their families to share their stories with us. I would like to extend a personal thanks to all of the contributors who spent months collaborating with me to make this project a reality.

I am equally grateful to Mary Kennan Herbert at Walker Publishing for her steady guidance and inspiration along the way. Many other people at Walker also spent time copyediting the manuscript and making valuable suggestions.

I would like to thank my friend and colleague Mary Thompson for leading me to this excellent opportunity. Steve Ross generously offered his time and years of experience in publishing. Pat and Bill Burleson and Tom Green opened their homes and offices to me, and Chris Astley contributed his talent as a photographer.

On the home front, I owe my gratitude to Dan White for his daily support and expert editing help. I also appreciate the unflagging interest and encouragement I received from my family.

Introduction

When people apply to medical school, they can become so focused on grades and test scores they lose sight of what they will actually be doing down the road, during their first year in practice. How can you tell if medicine is right for you? How do you know which specialty suits your personality?

My First Year as a Doctor offers readers a selection of essays by doctors in a broad range of specialties and geographical settings. In their own words, they talk about things many people never learn in medical school: How do you find time to have a family? What if I get sued? What about office politics? How do you tell family members when their loved one dies? How do you diagnose someone who doesn't speak your language?

This book contains conversations with an emergency physician in the South Bronx, a former coroner of Detroit, a family doctor in the heart of Appalachia, a plastic surgeon at Yale University, and a physician who develops drugs for the pharmaceutical industry, to name a few.

Despite their varied backgrounds, the doctors who contributed to this book had some common thoughts about their profession. Medicine offers an unusually satisfying combination of intellectual challenge and helping others. Dr. Mary Alfano, who has a family practice in Michigan, described it as a "tremendous detective game." Many came to the profession seeking prestige or respect, but they stayed because of the variety and contact with people from all walks of life. When Dr. Stephan Ariyan, a plastic surgeon from Connecticut, was in college he wanted a job that would allow him to look forward to Monday as much as the weekend. "I think medicine affords us that kind of pleasure," he says.

But every career choice has its pros and cons. Almost everyone in the book said they were unhappy with the way medicine is being changed from an art into a business by a growing health care bureaucracy. Some days they feel like they spend more time filling out forms than helping patients. Physicians also have to be willing to make a twenty-four-hour commitment. "When a patient is sick, they need you and they need you now," says Dr. Evan Provisor, a surgeon in Connecticut. Even when they are not on call, doctors often take cases home with them and worry about patients who aren't doing well. "Others rarely understand our long and frequently unpredictable hours," says Dr. Jacki Howitt, an obstetrician in New York. That can add up to strained relationships, and in some cases, burnout.

Another common theme that runs through the essays is the feeling of isolation that many young doctors encounter when they set out on their own after residency or fellowship. Ever since they began medical school, they were part of a group. If they had a question about what to do, a dozen classmates or the attending physician could help. Suddenly, they find themselves alone. "Without the security of my old academic setting, I felt like I was just going by the seat of my pants half the time," says Dr. David Preston, who spent his first year practicing internal medicine in a small town in Maine. That insecurity typically fades over time. "As with any job, the more you do it, the easier it gets," states Stan Thornton, an anesthesiologist in Texas. "I probably did anesthesia for one thousand different surgeries that year. After the first few hundred were under my belt, I was able to bolster my confidence."

Some physicians in the book pride themselves on being generalists. They chose areas like internal medicine and family practice, which emphasize patient education and preventive medicine. These physicians develop a close bond with patients because they see them on an ongoing basis. In her essay, "Medicine and Motherhood," Alfano describes how this makes her a better doctor.

When you have a history with a family that goes back a number of years like that, and you've been a major part of major events in their lives, you have a different relationship. Today, in my own practice, I have some families that have been with me now for ten or twelve years—I have delivered their babies, seen them through operations, and helped them cope with death. I've found that knowing people that well helps you put their problems in context.

In Preston's essay, "The Privilege of Listening," he also talks about the close bond between family doctor and patient. Some of his patients responded to him graciously. Others, like Hank, were not as easy to win over. The middle-aged man with a prison record was an inveterate smoker and alcoholic. Preston tried everything to help him change his habits but made little progress. In "Coming of Age in Appalachia," Dr. Steve Vogelsang encountered similar roadblocks in his community, where it is common for people to have "a six-to-eight-can-a-day cola habit" and smoke three packs a day. His patients often became ill with preventable conditions like coronary artery disease and hypertension. "There were times when these patients came in sick that I could have shook them and yelled, 'I told you so!'" Vogelsang says.

Preston and Dr. Erin Cardon, an internist who wrote "The Mind/Body Connection," both discovered that emotional issues and stress were often at the heart of the physical symptoms they saw day after day. "I chose primary care because I enjoy taking care of the whole person," Cardon says. To do so, generalists need a sound working knowledge of all the medical specialties.

In the opposite camp are the specialists, who have cultivated a deeper knowledge of one specific area. In "The Politics of Practice," Provisor describes his choice this way: "I chose my specialty because I like surgery. It's instant gratification. I don't like to sit around and wait for pills to work—to cut is to cure. You get to see the results of your work immediately. And it's a challenge. Surgery requires an enormous amount of judgment as well as technical skill."

People often ask Dr. Edward Dow, an oncologist, why he wanted to work with people who were dying of cancer. In "The Life in Death," he says, "I would find it much more depressing to be in a general medicine clinic where people have diabetes and alcoholism, things that you can treat effectively if the patient is motivated. But so many aren't." Dow enjoys working with patients who are highly motivated to do anything they can to prolong their life. "In oncology you're not dealing with neurotic diseases. You get the sense that you are dealing with real, concrete problems," Dow says. "If it's not there on the biopsy or the blood slide, the patient doesn't come to see me."

Specialists like Thornton, who does anesthesia for high-risk pediatric surgeries, have to think quickly on their feet. He says,

"People often compare doing anesthesia to being a pilot. . . . You have to have confidence in your decisions and act quickly." In both jobs, making the wrong decision can have disastrous consequences.

Most doctors work in a private practice office or a hospital, but some of the physicians in *My First Year as a Doctor* spend more time in the laboratory or the morgue. They show how medicine offers many options to new graduates who prefer to help others through research, not as clinicians.

While training in psychiatry, Dr. James Meador-Woodruff, who wrote "Mr. Jenkins's Holy Ghost," came to a crossroads. He wanted to help patients with schizophrenia. If he decided to go into a traditional practice, he would have a few ineffective medications to offer his patients. He decided to use his talents in a research setting instead. Since then, major breakthroughs in neurochemistry are helping researchers like Meador-Woodruff understand the brain better and improve quality of life for people with schizophrenia.

In hindsight, pathologist Dr. Werner Spitz also realized he was better suited to laboratory work than direct patient care. In his essay, "Memoir of a Forensic Pathologist," he acknowledges that pathology is grisly and gory, but doing autopsies doesn't bother him. "Somehow, your brain shifts gears. You don't experience all the nastiness because you do it day in and day out," he said. "If you don't think about what led up to a death, it becomes a thing, not a person anymore." Although they do not take care of patients in a traditional practice, pathologists play an important role by educating other physicians about the cause of disease, Spitz says.

Dr. Debra Williams chose an unusual career path after discovering the competitive world of academic medicine did not accommodate her need to raise a family. She gave up a faculty position at a prestigious university to help develop drugs in the pharmaceutical industry. She outlines the reason behind her change of heart in "Making the Switch to Pharmaceuticals."

> For a working mother, I had the best of all possible worlds. I had a full-time nanny living in, so I could leave the house at five in the morning if I wanted to and somebody would be taking care of the kids. My husband did all the cooking. Somebody came in to do the cleaning. I had the maximum support system, yet it was still impossible. The bottom line is the kids never saw me.

Other women in the book faced similar obstacles and came up with creative ways to cope with them. Alfano describes what it was like to be pregnant with her first child up until the last day of her residency. "I remember inserting the endotracheal tube to help this patient breathe, hoping nothing would happen because I was having contractions every three minutes," she says in her essay. She managed to breast-feed her baby, stay up with him at night, and still work full-time her first year in practice. Both Cardon and Dr. Susan Breen, an ophthalmologist in Massachusetts, opted to work part-time in a group practice so they could spend more time with their children. "It takes very careful planning to find or create a practice situation that can accommodate the tribulations of marriage and motherhood, but combining these roles can be a great source of joy," Breen says.

Working with patients from an unfamiliar culture provided a different type of challenge for physicians like Vogelsang, Dr. David Simenson, who works with migrant farm workers in California, and Dr. Allen Dobbs, who takes care of people on an Indian reservation in South Dakota. Simenson's patients often spoke different languages. He had to take their medical history, sort through their symptoms, and prescribe a treatment through one and sometimes two translators. To add to the confusion, some of the patients who emigrated from Mexico or Laos had their own set of folk remedies that were not familiar to Simenson. In "Cross-Cultural Medicine," Simenson tells what happened after he broke through the language barriers. "As I started medical practice, I began to develop stronger relationships with my patients," he says. "I better understood my patients—their different languages, dress, foods, and beliefs—and I saw many qualities to admire."

Vogelsang went through a similar change during his first year in one of the poorest counties in Kentucky. When he first arrived with the goal of bringing modern medical knowledge to poor patients, he met with resistance. Gradually, they began to accept him. "It is easy to deal with objective disease entities and not deal with the human lives made complicated by the disease. To do the latter requires that you get personal with your patients. Any personal relationship requires revealing something of yourself and stepping outside your clinical demeanor, something we are taught not to do in medical school."

Sometimes human lives are complicated not only by disease but also by social problems that make treating disease harder. In the South Bronx, where Dr. Brenda Merritt spent her first year in emergency medicine, few people have adequate health insurance. They often ignore their medical problems until they reach the critical point when they have to go to the hospital. In "The Front Lines of Emergency Medicine," Merritt tells what it's like to treat a homeless man for ulcers on his legs, only to have him return the next week with the same problem. "I did what I could for him, but I knew I was sending him back to the street," she says. Howitt, who specializes in problem pregnancies, sees many drug-addicted mothers in her practice. "Uncommon Heroes" describes one mother, Leticia, who decided to give up cocaine after Howitt and her colleagues showed her they cared about her in the clinic where she came for prenatal care.

The doctors in *My First Year as a Doctor* have many dramatic stories to tell, but each essay also contains practical advice and information. Stan Thornton talks about how to be prepared before you show up for your first day in the operating room. Susan Breen reminds you to find out what type of needles and other equipment you like the best so you can order them for your own office. Evan Provisor shows you how politics can sometimes get in the way of youthful ambition. And Mary Alfano offers an innovative way to solve child care problems when you could be called away any hour of the night.

My First Year as a Doctor will provide some compelling reading and may help you make a more informed choice about whether to become a doctor and what type of practice might be the most rewarding.

1

Coming of Age in Appalachia

 STEVE VOGELSANG

What a good thing, I thought, to come to eastern Kentucky and bring the poor of Appalachia the benefits of my newly acquired medical training—the latest treatments, medicines, and connections to the latest technology. Magoffin County is one of the poorest areas of the state: Its unemployment rate often tops 20 percent, over half its children live in poverty, and 60 percent of people over age twenty-five are high school dropouts. They needed me, I thought. What I didn't realize was that I needed them.

The greatest health problem here is lack of education, which translates into poor lifestyle choices. It is common to find a six-to-eight-can-a-day cola habit and twenty-pound buckets of lard on grocery shelves. The area has the highest smoking rate in the nation. It is no surprise that the most common conditions I see in the office are diabetes, coronary artery disease, emphysema, obesity, and hypertension.

As a result of my training, I had plenty of information to share.

Conversion to a healthy lifestyle would simply mean providing the less educated with the needed facts.

"How many packs a day do you smoke?"

"Oh, two or three, Doc."

I had just diagnosed the thin, wiry fifty-going-on-eighty-year-old man with pneumonia. I then launched into my "health risks of smoking" speech. He nodded respectfully with each point I made. I paused for his response.

"Well, Doc, you're right. But I just believe that when it's my time to go, I'm gonna go. There's just nothing a feller can do about that."

Hmmm, I thought, mountain fatalism; seems I had read about that somewhere. Multiply that conversation by a factor of several hundred and consider that I care for these people when they have strokes, heart attacks, or are diagnosed with lung cancer. I also often find myself tending to the grief of their families. That all adds up to a lot of frustration for a family physician, especially when you consider these are largely preventable conditions. There were times when these patients came in sick that I could have shook them and yelled, "I told you so!"

But with time my frustration, a symptom largely due to my own self-righteousness, mellowed into humility.

Each Christmas our clinic staff makes home visits to our neediest patients and delivers a small fruit basket. My family and I went to Emma's one special Christmas. Emma is a diabetic and badly needs to be on insulin. Multiple attempts by me, my staff, and the home health nurses failed to convince her of the importance of this. It seems a friend of hers who started insulin died shortly thereafter. Emma is convinced the same will happen to her.

She lives up a "holler" in a one-room shack that is solid and well insulated. It was built for her by a church group several winters ago when they found her living in an abandoned school bus.

As we entered the cabin that Christmas, the heat from the wood-burning stove was stifling. There were two small windows, three chairs, a kitchen table, a kerosene lamp, and a bed. Canned goods lined the walls, and clean clothes were off to the side on the floor. A small pile of wood was next to the potbellied stove (the rest she piles under the old school bus to keep it dry). There was no electricity, no refrigerator, and no indoor plumbing. At sixty-eight years old she still cuts her own firewood. This situation is not the norm in eastern Kentucky, but it's not uncommon either.

Emma's way is deliberate, quiet, and peaceful. As we exchanged the usual initial pleasantries, I couldn't help but pity her. My mind raced through the improvements we could make to this hut to make it more livable. The chance for the question came.

"Emma, how would you like to have some electricity put in?"

"Oh, I don't think so. . . . I don't need the bill, my kerosene lamp provides enough light. I keep my food cool outside," she said. "I'm happy enough with what I have."

Our conversation turned to world events. She is an avid reader of the newspaper and her Bible. She knows what's out there. She knows what the world has to offer and adeptly uses current events to demonstrate the wisdom of the Bible. It is her source of truth and she sees it clearly within the simple life she has chosen. I couldn't help but respect her and be humbled by her.

With humility comes acceptance. With my acceptance of them, my patients began to let me into their lives, not just their medical problems. The former deeply affects the latter. With insight into a person's life, treatment of a problem becomes more effective.

Flora was sixty years old and suffered from angina and severe arthritis of both her shoulders. We tried many medications for her arthritis but they never seemed to help. She came in one day when her pain was particularly severe. As I examined her, she nearly screamed when I attempted to lift her arms above her head.

I didn't know what else to do for her and I guess it showed on my face.

"Doctor, I feel like I can trust you," Flora said.

She proceeded to tell me about how she cared for her retarded daughter Rita who had cerebral palsy, was wheelchair bound, and weighed over 220 pounds. She had to lift her often as she transferred her to chairs and the bed and while using bathroom facilities. "I never felt like I could ask for help because I'm afraid I would lose Rita," Flora said. She then explained how she feared the Department of Social Services would take her daughter from her if she wasn't able to care for her. I convinced her that this certainly was not the case. With that, home health nurses and aides began to help Flora care for Rita five days a week. Flora's arthritis improved far beyond what any medicine alone could have accomplished for her. The success from this treatment didn't so much come from my training as it did from my friendship.

It is easy to deal with objective disease entities and not deal with the human lives made complicated by disease. To do the latter requires that you get personal with your patients. Any personal relationship requires revealing something of yourself and stepping outside your clinical demeanor, something we are taught not to do in medical school.

But it was unavoidable after spending time here with the people of eastern Kentucky. They have a way of disarming you with their unabashed realism, gentleness, and patience.

I soon found myself taking my kids to Ruthie's house to make apple butter. Ruthie was a tough, kind mountain woman with a terminal heart disease. She loved teaching us the mountain lore and ways of her youth. I had the privilege of getting to know her most valued treasures: her faith, her husband and family, and her neighbors. And when it came time for her to die, she clapped her hands and sang. To the nurses, I'm sure it seemed like the onset of delirium in her final moments. But to me, the meaning was crystal clear. She was about to meet her Creator, the source of her life's joy and treasures.

It was a good thing I came to eastern Kentucky. I rarely suffer from burnout anymore. Here, I learned that caring about people is the best medicine for my patients and for me.

> *Steve Vogelsang is a family physician and medical director of a family medical center in Kentucky.*

2

The Mind/Body Connection

 ERIN CARDON

One of my patients came to my office complaining of chronic headaches that sometimes kept her in bed all day. I later found out she worked in a clerical job where she felt a lot of pressure but received very little recognition from her boss. I also took care of an older woman who suddenly became very sick with cancer about four months after her spouse of fifty-two years passed away. Another patient was waking up with night sweats and heart palpitations. During subsequent visits, she revealed that she was married to an alcoholic who emotionally abused her.

Partway through my first year as a general internist who specializes in women's health, I began to notice a pattern. My patients showed me how our mental status can govern our physical being. One of the most common examples of this is the case of nerves people get before taking a big test or standing in front of a crowd to give a speech. The heart rate speeds, the hands and face sweat, the appetite diminishes, the skin flushes, and the intestines may cramp. This is a short-lived experience. But what happens to the body when the mind is dealt a stress that doesn't ease? What is the interplay of mind and body? Science is only beginning to reveal the neurochemical, immunological, and hormonal factors behind this phenomenon. In my practice of medicine, I was being asked to deal with the mind/body relationship on a daily basis.

During my first year in practice, I was astounded by the number of women who were seeking help for a complex of symptoms known as panic attack. These symptoms include shortness of breath, chest pressure, lightheadedness, trembling, nausea, vertigo, and finally, an overwhelming fear of losing control. I was seeing two or three new patients a week in varying stages of panic disorder. Many of these women had seen a number of specialists before they came to me. They may have seen a cardiologist for the chest pains, an ear, nose, and throat specialist for the vertigo, or a pulmonary specialist for their shortness of breath. The patients often had several tests and were told everything was normal. Discouraged and feeling dismissed, they continued to suffer with their symptoms.

Nobody ever sat down with these patients to figure out what was going on and put the whole picture together. Once I spent some time clarifying their symptoms, the diagnosis was usually very straightforward. During the interview, I helped the patients identify the source of the stress that was driving the panic disorder. For many women, this may have been the stress of dealing with an unhappy marriage, a job change, or memories of a past rape or incest that had begun to bubble to the surface of their consciousness. The reasons were as numerous as the individual patients. These patients were greatly relieved to learn that treatments were available to them. I had a lot of success helping these women control their symptoms with a multidisciplinary approach of medication, psychotherapy, and behavior modification.

Because of the demands of my own patient population, I felt

there must be other people who were also needlessly suffering. I wrote an article pertaining to panic attack in our health center's community publication. As a follow-up, I gave a public seminar on the topic. During the first several days that this announcement ran, our center received over one hundred calls from people who wanted to attend. At the seminar, we gave participants a lot of references on the subject and advised them to see a general internist who could rule out other medical disorders and confirm the diagnosis. Many of the people who came to the conference sought treatment at our center. The therapists who shared an office with us agreed to lead a behavioral therapy group for people with panic disorder. Within a year, some of these women were living more happy and productive lives. That was one of the most gratifying experiences I had my first year in practice.

I chose primary care because I enjoy taking care of the whole person. Internists assimilate the physical symptoms with the psychosocial setting and provide comprehensive care. To do this, they need to have a sound knowledge of basic science and the different subspecialties of medicine. Diseases may fall into distinct categories and classifications, but people do not. Often, a patient's problems overlap many disciplines. Like the women who came to me with panic disorder, people sometimes need one complete physician rather than myriad specialists. Physicians who view patients as a disease that needs to be fixed get bored. I discovered that seeing patients as individuals and treating them holistically is much more interesting.

Thinking about the way the mind affects the body is an integral part of that process. Unless you look at the underlying life stresses, you are simply putting a Band-Aid on the problem. That is partly why I chose to specialize in stress-related health problems that tend to affect women in greater numbers. I feel we have a lot more to learn about the physical and psychological forces behind panic disorder, irritable bowel, premenstrual syndrome, headaches, and other illnesses triggered by stress.

As an internist, I greatly enjoy my role as a diagnostician. I have cultivated an intuitive sense about illness, which is continually being fine-tuned. Listening to people talk about emotional issues for eight or ten hours a day can be very draining. But it is only in being attentive to the patient, truly listening and ultimately caring about what is being said, that the art of diagnosis reveals itself. The physician must remain disciplined in order to pay attention to what the patient is saying and then use judgment at least as much as technology to arrive at a diagnosis.

After I arrive at a diagnosis, the next step is to allow the patient to become a partner in deciding how to confirm the diagnosis and what course of treatment to follow. One of my primary roles as an internist is to educate patients about their illness. I typically discuss preventive measures, the origins of the disease, and both the benefits and possible side effects of the medication they may use. In doing this, I ask that the patients become responsible for their health. When patients are well informed, they are more compliant and interested in maintaining their health. In internal medicine there is little immediate gratification. But when I can help a patient decide to stop smoking or lose twenty pounds by exercising, I feel I've accomplished something important.

In the future, medicine will rely on the general internist more to provide basic comprehensive and preventive care and to be the "gatekeepers" who decide the need for specialty care. It will also be interesting to see how things change as more women enter medicine. There will probably be more generalists and primary care physicians as a result of this trend. More salaried positions in HMOs and large group practices will appeal to women who also want to be mothers. In that setting, they would not have to be on call every other weekend like they would if they went into private practice. I was lucky enough to find an arrangement where I shared a position with another woman who was having twins so we could both work part-time and raise our children.

I decided to go into medicine as a career because it combined my love of science and working with people. Today, I see it as more than an occupation. It is an extension of my ability to communicate well and my desire to help others. Being a physician has given me a unique chance to explore what life is all about. In doing so, I have enriched my own life. Practicing internal medicine has given me a great opportunity for self-discovery, and I am continually learning how to become a better listener and caregiver for my fellow human beings. My personal life experience as a wife, mother, and daughter—and in dealing with illness and death in my own family—has contributed to my becoming a whole physician, one who can listen attentively with both empathy and knowledge.

Erin Cardon is a general internist at a women's wellness center in Connecticut.

3

The Politics of Practice

 EVAN PROVISOR

During the last few months of my general surgery residency in Providence, Rhode Island, I saw an ad placed by a surgeon in a small town in Connecticut who was looking for a young physician to join his practice. I called him and we agreed to meet for an interview.

My wife, Pam, and I piled into our beat-up old 1974 Gremlin (affectionately nicknamed "the pregnant roller skate") and drove into the rural, New England town in the middle of a snowstorm. I took in the traditional town green, with its stone clock tower and old clapboard homes, and thought how charming everything looked. My wife loved it, too.

Fred, the surgeon who interviewed me, was an older man in his sixties who wore a western-style tie around his neck. He showed me around the small community hospital across the street from his office, and we had lunch at a little restaurant nearby. I took the job when he offered it, without giving the decision much thought. Fred seemed like a nice guy who was practicing good medicine in the community and the town looked like the perfect place to bring up our children, so I signed the one-year employment contract he had drawn up for me.

As the year unfolded, I discovered that I was seventh in a long line of associates who had all left because he offered them promises of partnership in the practice that never materialized. I started to wish I had asked around more about Fred's track record before I signed on with him. That first year also taught me that politics can sometimes get in the way of giving patients the best possible care in communities where physicians are entrenched in turf wars.

When I first started out with Fred, I spent a lot of time assisting him in the operating room. I was young and gung-ho. I didn't mind working extra hours, so I offered to take over for Fred the nights he was on call at the emergency room. It was a good way to build up my practice base, and within a few months, I was fairly busy with my own patients.

About a month after I arrived—on my birthday—I got called to the emergency room because of a man who was bleeding from his neck. He was using a chain saw that kicked back and sliced him right at the base of his neck down through his collarbone. He was bleeding to death. I ran from the office over to the emergency room, quickly put pressure on the wound, and took him off to the operating room. I was able to stop the bleeding and save his life. The thing I remember about him was that he was somewhat of an ingrate. Sure, he was glad to be alive, but he was really angry because he had cut one of the nerves that goes to the diaphragm on one side, so his breathing capacity was limited. I was taken aback. I thought he should have been grateful that he was alive. It made me realize that people's expectations are often greater than what you can deliver. Even when you save someone's life, it might not be good enough.

Not everything was life or death my first year. In the office I spent a lot of time removing warts and taking off various lumps and bumps. The first patient I saw my first day of practice had varicose veins. I've come to despise the surgery for this; it's boring, tedious, and calls for very tiny incisions and a lot of cutting and sewing. I did a lot of what we call bread-and-butter surgery that year—gallbladders, colon removals, breast surgery.

I chose my specialty because I like surgery. It's instant gratification. I don't like to sit around and wait for pills to work—to cut is to cure. You get to see the results of your work immediately. And it's a challenge. Surgery requires an enormous amount of judgment as well as technical skill. You have to know your anatomy well. You have to know when to change your tactic and how to deal with unforeseen consequences. For example, one time I operated on a woman for what I thought was acute appendicitis. When I made the incision and opened her up, it turned out that she had an inflamed gallbladder, so I took out both her appendix and her gallbladder.

On most days, I would get up and go into the hospital around seven-thirty to see patients on rounds and then spend the rest of the morning in the operating room. Surgery was usually finished by around one o'clock, and I would go over to the office and have lunch. Between two and five o'clock, I saw patients in the office. Most people came in for follow-up visits after surgery, to prepare for an operation, or for office surgery.

I knew that it was important to communicate with my patients because most malpractice lawsuits are brought by people who are angry. If someone had a problem or a complication, I would try to see them through it and make sure they knew I cared about them. Before a surgery, I spent at least half of the visit educating the patient so he or she would understand what to expect and what the potential complications were.

In between patients, I tried to update charts and get all my paperwork done. Before I went home for the day, I would go back to the hospital for my last set of rounds between five and six o'clock. But even when I was home, the workday didn't end. The phone sometimes rang all night with calls from patients who had questions or unexpected complications. If I got a call that there had been a bad automobile accident and the patient was having internal bleeding, that was it. I had to go. Some nights there weren't many calls, but if I had a sick patient who wasn't doing well, I would sit and worry about the person. You can never just turn it off when you come home.

One thing that was a godsend that year was my wife. She is a surgical intensive care nurse, and because of that she understood my schedule. She understood that when a patient is sick, they need you and they need you now. One of the other surgeons had a wife who could not accept that. If they had plans to go out and he got called, she was very upset. They have subsequently divorced.

As it got closer to the holidays, I started to wonder when Fred was going to give me my Christmas bonus. He did finally give me a bonus, but it didn't buy many presents. It was a fruitcake. I was learning and gaining experience each day I worked for Fred, so I didn't complain. Besides, I had a new project that had captured my interest.

I was putting together a proposal to have the local hospital open a new $15,000 vascular surgery laboratory that would evaluate patients with vascular diseases like arteriosclerosis, poor circulation, and stroke. During my training at Brown University I learned some techniques that weren't being done locally. I had hopes of making vascular surgery a major part of the institution so the hospital could use the specialty to draw in new patients.

As a medical student, I never thought about the politics of practice. I thought that if you were a good doctor and you practiced good medicine, then your patients would like you and you would do well. But it wasn't that simple, I found out. At the time, there were two political factions in town. One was the group of physicians at a large multispecialty clinic, and the other was the independent doctors who were not associated with the clinic. It was clinic versus nonclinic. There was a lot of rivalry between the two groups and competition for patients. Being employed by a nonclinic physician, I was immediately drawn into that conflict. I had no desire to get embroiled in politics the first year I got there, but there was no avoiding it.

Unfortunately, because I was not on the clinic staff and most of the hospital budget committee was, my vascular laboratory project was blocked because of politics. There was no way they were going to allow the expenditure for this laboratory. They didn't want to see a nonclinic doctor do too well. It was a setback. I didn't give up, but it did dash my hopes. I realized you don't have a lot of power your first year of practice. And cutting-edge ideas are not always appreciated. I kept fighting for it and finally got it a number of years later. By then, however, it cost $30,000.

My first year working in Fred's practice was almost over when I made a discreet inquiry about a clause in my contract that said I could get a bonus for exceptional performance. I worked hard and generated a lot of extra revenue for him that year, so I had no doubt that he would give it to me. When I asked him about it, he told me that yes, I had generated a lot of revenue, but because he had let me take his ER call, that was work he would have otherwise done himself. Therefore I wasn't entitled to a bonus. I started to realize my association with Fred had probably been a mistake.

Around the same time, a good friend of mine who joined a practice with a local obstetrician came up against a different problem with his employment contract. When he wanted to leave after a year, he discovered that his employer put in a clause that prevented him from setting up a competing practice in the same community for the next three years. Even though he and his wife bought a house and wanted to raise their kids there, he ended up moving to Virginia so he could set up his own practice. Fortunately, my contract didn't have one of those noncompetition clauses. If it did, I would never have known to look for it and I would have been in the same boat.

A few months before my one-year anniversary, Fred came to my office with a legal document. He said he was ready to retire and wanted me to buy his practice. I was surprised, because he had led me to believe that I would become his partner at the end of the year. My understanding and his understanding of our future together were different.

I didn't want to take over his practice because his terms for a buyout were not acceptable to me. Aside from purchasing the assets—office space, furniture, equipment, and the accounts receivable—he wanted me to pay him a $100,000 goodwill fee for the privilege of taking over the patients he had cultivated over the years. But without him there, his practice was not worth very much to me. Patients tend to be very selective about their surgeons. Reputation is important. If he retired, there was no guarantee that his patients would automatically come to me. They had a choice of three other surgeons in town at the time. So I told him, "I'm sorry, I can't do this," and gave him notice that I was going to terminate my contract in ninety days.

Needless to say, Fred was angry. He felt he had given me my start by letting me practice on "his" patients and I let him down. He thought I was an ingrate. When my contract ran out, I decided to stay in the community and set up a practice on my own.

Going to work for someone else has the advantage that you don't have to worry about setting up an office, ordering supplies, hiring staff, and meeting a payroll. All the business aspects of running a practice don't exist. The downside is that you don't have quite the same economic incentive; no matter how hard you work, it doesn't necessarily mean you're going to make more money.

Very few doctors set up practice on their own right out of residency. It's a big hassle with a lot of insecurity and no guaranteed income. There was no way I could have afforded to do that out of residency; I had to start making payments on my educational loans. I was also very unsophisticated coming out of residency. I knew nothing about private practice. After I got there, I learned some of the questions I should have asked. I would have talked more to my employer's former associates, colleagues, and peers. I would have asked: How good is this person technically? How good is his or her reputation? What has the track record been of other people who have associated with this person? Is this person ethical?

You also want to make sure the person is board certified and a member in good standing of local medical societies and professional organizations. It's a good idea to ask about the political climate, too. How well do doctors in the area work together? Do they share cases or do they compete with one another?

Most people choose a spouse with more care than they choose a practice, but you will spend more time with your partner than your wife or husband. I may have been frustrated with my employment situation that first year, but I discovered that being your own boss isn't all it's cracked up to be either. During the following year, when I opened up my solo practice, I learned that no one has a boss as mean, as demanding, and as unmerciful as the person who is self-employed.

Evan Provisor is a general surgeon in Connecticut.

4

The Life in Death

 E D W A R D   D O W

It was an unusually clear day in downtown Seattle, so I could watch the sun go down over the Olympic Mountains and the waters of Puget Sound. In the sunset, the skyscrapers glowed with a surreal orange light. I was watching from a conference room at the hospital where I was doing an oncology fellowship. It seemed strange to be surrounded by so much natural beauty in the middle of so much aching, man-made sadness. I wasn't able to enjoy the view much. I was mediating a tense family conference over a dying young woman named Sandra.

Sandra, who was in her thirties, had recurrent Hodgkin's lymphoma. Everything had been done to stop it, including a bone marrow transplant. She was later readmitted after she developed pneumonia and her condition deteriorated. She was now in a coma, breathing mechanically on a respirator, with no sign of life. After I explained to the family that Sandra had a slim chance of survival, we all got together to decide whether or not to take her off life support. Three or four different forces were competing for control in the room.

Sandra's mother, Pauline, had a strong, controlling personality. She was extremely involved in Sandra's care, staying by her bed day and night. Although Sandra was an adult, Pauline made all the decisions for her. She argued strongly in favor of keeping her daughter alive. She was pitted against Sandra's husband, Jim, who actually had legal power of attorney. He felt it would be wrong to draw out her life any longer. Jim, who had been separated from Sandra for several years and had a child with her, flew in from Wyoming for the family meeting. He made Pauline out to be a dragon-lady. He blamed her for coming between him and Sandra. Pauline, on the other hand, hinted to me that Jim was a good-for-nothing who treated her daughter badly.

Also in the room were Sandra's father, Ted, a preacher who was no longer married to Pauline; Pauline's second husband, John; and their family minister, Ron. These three men brought their own agendas to the table. Negotiating a compromise in this meeting was tough. It was like brokering the Middle East peace talks. It turned out that my greatest ally was Sandra's husband, Jim. He gave the impression of being an uneducated working guy who liked to party, but he rose to the fore. I was amazed and grateful to him. He realized that Sandra was now just a lifeless form being kept alive by a tangle of tubes and machines. After Pauline made her pitch for keeping Sandra alive, Jim began to speak.

"I really think it's inhumane to let her go on like this," he said.

Jim looked straight at Pauline. "I know you and I don't get along. I don't know if I even like you, but I love Sandra," he said. "I thought it over and I've got to do what's right."

Since Jim and Sandra had never actually divorced, he had the legal right to make the decision. But to my delight and surprise, he wanted it to be a group decision. "I think we've all got to agree here and now to do this," he said.

As the family members thought it over in tense silence, they began to realize their differences were kind of petty. They were all there on behalf of this young woman and yet they couldn't love one another. I think the conflict started to seem insignificant to them.

Mary Ann, the sister of Ted's second wife, was also in the room. I noticed she wore a large crucifix and wondered what her thoughts would be. She had been quiet during the whole meeting, but suddenly she spoke up.

"I had a similar experience with my mother when she had lung cancer two years ago," she said.

The tears started rolling down her face as she told the story of how she decided to take her mother off life support. "I believe in God and I believe that life is a sacred thing," she said. "My mother was not alive. Her body was there, but her soul was already in heaven. I told them to shut the machines off because I wanted to end her suffering and give her some peace," she said.

Mary Ann's story sort of got people to agree to let Sandra go, but they wouldn't have arrived at the decision without Jim's powerful appeal. They had painted an unsavory picture of Jim, but he turned out to be a pretty strong human being. They struggled and finally came together; that was the beautiful thing about it.

During that family meeting, I remember looking at the corporate office buildings across the street and thinking, "I guess this is why I do what I do instead of being a businessman or a lawyer." I was dealing with pure humanity in that conference room. In oncology, you see people grappling in very real terms with love, death, commitment, and God versus no God. I found that I enjoyed working with families like Sandra's, sorting through all the layers of psychology and helping them cope with the death of a loved one.

They always say tragedy brings out the best or the worst in a person and I found that to be true. If a person is a real jerk, getting sick is usually going to intensify that. It's the same with families. If a family is very dysfunctional and a member gets sick, it's going to put an even worse spin on it. Sometimes more than what is appropriate gets done for the patient because things are so chaotic and the family can't agree.

People who meet me often ask, "How can you work with cancer patients? It must be so depressing!" I would find it much more depressing to be in general medicine where people have diabetes and alcoholism—things that you can treat effectively if the patient is motivated. But so many people aren't. To me, treating some patient who had a stroke because he didn't take his blood pressure pills would be much more depressing than what I do. My patients may die, but at least they've done everything they can. They not only follow my instructions to the letter but they also go and find out things on their own. They're much more motivated. In oncology you're not dealing with neurotic diseases. You get the sense that you are dealing with real, concrete problems. If it's not there on the biopsy or the blood slide, the patient doesn't come to see me.

The art of being a good clinician is sizing up the person intellectually, spiritually and psychologically. The key is to be truthful. The truth may be bad news, but at least the burden of ignorance is lifted. You have to be careful about giving too much information all at once or the patient could be overloaded. You might have to let the truth out in little bits. For many of my patients, there's a big state of denial at first. People don't want to believe they have cancer or any other serious malady. You must never take all hope away. You have to convince your patients that no matter what, you're going to be there to give them comfort and alleviate their suffering. You must establish that you're their advocate.

As an oncologist, I see people die two or three times a month. In a few cases, when I have had a close bond with the patients, I had a hard time with their deaths. You have to take it home with you once in a while and it can wear on your mind. I started my training at Tufts University before going to Seattle for a year. I had a patient at Tufts who developed a rare and fatal leukemia.

The patient, Rick, was about forty. He was an extremely nice guy who was very close to his wife, Jane. They had a beautiful child named Jamie. I remember how she was sitting on his lap when I told him that his myelofibrosis had turned into leukemia. I just about lost it. Over the next few months, I grew attached to Rick and his family. He was a very gentle, kind man who told great stories. His work brought him to the outdoors and he had a love of nature. You could see that he was a sweet and devoted husband and loving father. I wondered what it would be like for his family after he was gone.

The Christmas before Rick died, his wife made a batch of homemade jelly and gave it to all the nurses and doctors who took care of him. I kept that jar of jelly on my shelf for a year or so, in his memory. One day I was feeling kind of blue, so I decided to take it down and eat a meal in honor of him. I wanted to honor him because he faced his end with such dignity, humility, and calmness. He possessed an inner peace and strength that few ever do. That night, thoughts of that gentle man cheered me and made me realize my troubles at the moment were merely surmountable obstacles.

When I returned to Boston to work at Massachusetts General Hospital, I took care of a therapist named Jonathan who had a similar form of leukemia. Jonathan knew the prognosis was bad, but he was a very tough guy mentally. He told us he wanted to pursue aggressive chemotherapy. I enjoyed working with Jonathan. He reminded me a little of Woody Allen with his fatalistic sense of humor, but his dread was very real. His wife, Cheryl, was a wonderful woman, too. They had no children, but they had an extremely close, supportive circle of friends. They were all very nice people. Part of the time I was treating Jonathan, he continued to see his patients whenever he felt well enough to go into his office.

It was around December when Jonathan started feeling worse, and we admitted him to the hospital. He was not responding well to the chemotherapy, and was in pretty bad shape. The other doctor in charge of his care felt we should not resuscitate him if he started to slip any further. He didn't want to see the patient suffer. My feeling was that if we were going to be aggressive, we should be consistent about it. This was a guy who wanted us to push aggressively, and I wanted to continue in that aggressive mode out of respect to his and his wife's wishes. At the behest of my superior, I eventually convinced Cheryl to agree to discontinue treatment and forgo aggressive resuscitation should he continue to fail.

I felt terrible about this because I knew he had put a lot of trust in me. Did I violate my patient's trust or had I allowed myself to be set up for this? If I respected his wishes would I indeed be doing bad medicine by prolonging suffering? Jonathan died a few days later. It was a snowy Saturday morning. I wasn't on call that day, but Cheryl called me from the hospital and told me.

"Are you coming in?" she asked.

I said I would even though a real blizzard was raging outside. Cheryl didn't have a big family. I was as much a part of her support system as anybody, so I felt I should be there for her. When

I got to the hospital, I found Cheryl and gave her a hug. "Was he comfortable?" I asked.

"As much as possible, I guess," she said.

"He didn't suffer long," I said. "He got to see his patients and have some good times outside the hospital."

I found that when dealing with death constantly, you can become desensitized, which is different from being insensitive. You can empathize and be sensitive when patients need support, but you can't let it derail you emotionally because of your own survival and the need to function for your other patients. You can't always take off for an afternoon to go cry by the riverside when you lose a patient you cared about, because you've got three other patients who are walking disasters back in the clinic.

A lot of frustration builds up when people aren't doing well despite your best efforts. Surgeons sometimes have it easier—they can come into the operating room, remove a tumor, and walk away without having much contact with the patient. I'm the guy who's left with the long-term job, seeing the patient through to the end. My satisfaction comes from the little things I can do for patients: gaining their trust, removing doubt, alleviating their suffering, and helping them come to terms with an intolerable situation.

Although there are some sorely tragic moments, I find oncology to be a rewarding field. Seeing young patients like Sandra, Rick, and Jonathan struggle with their mortality has changed my outlook on life. It's made me realize that the time to start enjoying life is right now. When I decided to go to medical school, I was upholding a family tradition. My father is a doctor and my mother's father was a doctor. My mother had been a nurse and her mother was a nurse. There was always that message that the noblest thing you could do was to pursue a medical career. I found out medicine also involves a lot of delayed gratification. We enter the marketplace and begin earning a living a lot later than our peers. We put a lot of life's decisions on hold. I've always had this ascetic mentality, thinking everyone else got to go to the beach or the party, but I couldn't because I had to study so I could get into medical school or I had to stay late at the hospital because I was in medical school. Lately, I've made a point to go to the beach or go skiing on weekends when I can. It's starting to make me think about valuing life, making some time for myself and having good times while I can enjoy them. I don't want to find myself on the other end of the IV needle someday, wishing I had done things differently.

Edward Dow is a staff hematologist/oncologist at a hospital in Boston.

5

Plastic Surgery: More than Noses and Breasts

 STEPHAN ARIYAN

For as long as I can remember back into my childhood, I have always wanted to be a doctor. By the time I was a first-year medical student, I knew I wanted to be a surgeon. At the time, I couldn't think of anything less interesting than plastic surgery. I mistakenly thought the field dealt only with frivolous cosmetic surgery. Early on, I was attracted to the idea of operating on hearts. As I proceeded through medical school, however, I also became interested in neurosurgery. This fine, delicate type of surgery that could remove tumors without damaging the brain fascinated me.

After spending time observing both types of surgery in the operating room, I settled on a career in cardiac surgery. I began my internship in the late 1960s. That was an exciting time. New heart-lung machines were being developed that allowed for more extensive bypass operations on the heart. I thought I had truly found the excitement I was looking for until I made an unsettling observation: All the best chief residents at the institution were going for further training in plastic surgery. My curiosity got the better of me. Either there was something wrong with these talented surgeons or I had missed something in my medical training. I decided to spend more time in this area to see what it was all about.

Suddenly, I realized plastic surgery included not only cosmetic surgery but also a whole new arena of reconstructive surgery that I had not been aware of. I saw restorative surgery for children born with birth defects such as cleft palates and absent ears, fingers, or hands. Some of the operations filled holes left by cancer surgery and erased scars from severe burns. Other surgeries restored function to the muscles, tendons, and nerves of hands that were injured at work or play.

The following year I was selected to serve in the U.S. Navy. This interrupted my surgical training, but it also gave me time to think about my career path. I spent my first year on an aircraft carrier in the Vietnam conflict. While stationed in San Diego the second year, I was able to do some research on kidney transplants at the University of California. I discovered that it was plastic surgeons who first studied the problem of organ transplant rejection. Later that year, I had the chance to spend a day with Dr. Joseph Murray, a plastic surgeon from Boston who performed the first human kidney transplant operation. On the same trip, I also met Dr. Thomas Kriszek, who was the chief of plastic surgery at Yale Medical Center. He was the most exciting teacher I had ever come across. Inspired by this experience, I decided on my career: plastic and reconstructive surgery.

When my two years in the navy were over, I finished my general surgery training at Yale and also began my residency there in plastic surgery. Although many of us select the areas of medicine we go into based on interests or personality traits, it seems that individual mentors also have a strong impact on many physicians. I became interested in plastic surgery because I admired those capable chief residents at UCLA and had the opportunity to meet Drs. Murray and Kriszek.

After my residency, I intended to move back to California, but my mentor, Dr. Kriszek, asked me to stay on at Yale and join the faculty. It was an offer I could not turn down. At Yale, I had access to research opportunities and clinical activities with respected and accomplished physicians that would not be available to me if I went into private practice.

One such opportunity arose when a woman was referred to me during my first year as an attending surgeon at Yale. This patient used to work in the watch factories that thrived in Connecticut between the 1920s and 1940s. In those days, radioactive material was used to paint numbers and dots on the watch dials so they would glow in the dark. This patient and her co-workers used to lick the tips of their paintbrushes to make a fine point. After years of performing this task, this woman had absorbed radium into her body, which deposited in her bones. This type of low-dose radioactivity usually does very little harm. But in her case, it was a different story. The radium was deposited in the bones and sinus cavities around her face. The trapped air in the sinuses mixed with the radium and turned into radioactive gas. This chronic exposure to low-level radioactivity irritated the cells lining her sinuses. Eventually, they began to produce cancerous growths.

The woman was referred to me for cancer in the sinuses around her eye. It destroyed her eye and the bones surrounding it. I would have to surgically remove the bone on her forehead, the undersurface of her brain, her eye, and her cheekbones. The procedure would leave a large hole that would make reconstruction very difficult. Fortunately, the patient refused the operation, which gave me time to consider a possible solution. I knew that sooner or later she would be coming back with pain and perhaps some bleeding that would require an operation. I needed to be prepared for reconstruction.

I decided to go to the autopsy room to look for different tissues I could use. There was a popular flap at the time that used the skin and fat of the chest for reconstructing many parts of the face and neck. Unfortunately, it didn't have enough bulk or tissue to fill such a large hole. I decided to look in the autopsy room again to see if I could bring the chest muscle along with the flap for added bulk.

In the process, I discovered that the muscle had its own separate blood supply. It could be moved to any part of the head or neck while the blood vessels were still intact. This would greatly reduce the chance of infection after the flap was attached to a new location. My observation contradicted what I learned in anatomy. I was taught that the blood supply to this major chest muscle came up through a deeper layer of muscles. Instead, it had its own direct blood supply. As I expected, the patient had further problems with pain and bleeding and returned to have the operation. I now had the opportunity to use this muscle and soft tissue from the chest wall to fill in the section that was removed.

Coincidentally, I had been asked by the American College of Surgeons to make a surgical film for its annual meeting. Each year, about ten people demonstrate a surgical technique on film to help other physicians with continuing education. When the woman from the watch factory came back for this operation, I called the film crew to ask if they would be willing to film this unusual technique. They agreed. The operation turned out to be a success and we captured the first procedure of this kind on film. We repeated the operation on several other patients with similar cancers and it turned out to be very reliable and versatile. It could be used in just about any part of the head and neck area. It also tended to heal without infections and complications.

I think the most compelling part of my first year was this patient who prompted our search for this new technique. It allowed
us to treat most cancers in the head and neck region with a single
operation, and patients recovered after seven to ten days. The old
method required two or three different surgeries, and patients typically stayed in the hospital for two or three months. This case
changed what we were eventually able to do for thousands of
similar patients throughout the world.

I was very lucky to have the institution, facilities, and support
that allowed me to do this research and develop the idea of using
chest muscles for reconstruction. Often physicians in private practice have ideas they want to explore but do not have the time or
facilities to pursue them further. I think my academic environment
has a lot to do with how I developed as a professional. Once
people are given the encouragement and support, they become
most productive.

As a medical student, I mistakenly thought I had more to offer
medicine than taking care of noses and breasts. After taking care
of all kinds of deformities, I realized this was a very unfair and
biased viewpoint. I learned that appearance is very important to
patients. For example, if a girl was burned as a child, those scars
would be disturbing to her through adolescence and adulthood.
Everyone can understand that. But patients who feel they have an
abnormal appearance are equally important. A child who grows
up with prominent ears, a man who is concerned about a hump
on his nose, or a woman who is self-conscious about being very
large-breasted also deserve our attention. We need to be less judg-
mental about patients and more understanding.

Still, it is important to determine whether a patient requesting
cosmetic procedures has inappropriate expectations. Sometimes
people who do not feel good about themselves have the miscon-

ception that their life will change if they have a perfect nose. These patients need to be discouraged from having the operation because they are destined to be unhappy regardless of the outcome.

A man came to me in the plastic surgery clinic at the nearby veteran's hospital. He requested a facelift because his skin was sagging. On the surface, he seemed to be an appropriate candidate. This patient, however, came into the office with cellophane tape on each side of his face, pulling the skin up to his ear. He said he wanted to demonstrate the improvement this operation could make in his appearance. This automatically raised a red flag in my mind. Furthermore, I wondered why this man, who lived in New Jersey, traveled to Connecticut when there were several other VA hospitals along the way. He responded that if he was going to have a facelift, he wanted to go to the best. He figured Yale was the best. It's easy to fall into the trap when someone is using flattery, but I could not help but feel that something was wrong. I explained to him that I needed to have some more visits before I made the final arrangements. I also suggested that he have a psychiatric evaluation to determine whether the operation would be appropriate in his case. This did not seem to distrub the patient in any way.

About an hour after the man left, two hospital security officers came to me to ask if I had seen the patient. They specifically asked if the patient needed any urgent medical care. I was curious to find out what happened. They explained that this man went from my office to the chief of staff's office to demand that he be taken care of immediately. As a veteran, he deserved better treatment, he said. He wanted to be hospitalized right away. He had been abusive and physically threatening. As I suspected, he had some psychiatric problems, but they were subtle and hard to pick up in one short office visit where he was on his best behavior. Obviously, the reasons the patient wanted cosmetic surgery were inappropriate at the time.

Medicine has changed a great deal since I started to practice. The delight of medicine is that every morning that I get up, I still look forward to the day. I remember when I was in college, I wanted eventually to have a job that would allow me to look forward to Monday when Sunday ended as much as I had looked forward to the weekend. I think medicine affords us that kind of pleasure. Every few years I see surveys that have interviews with physicians to show the satisfaction levels in different specialties. Invariably, plastic surgery has a high satisfaction rate. Part of this may have to do with the variety of cases this specialty offers.

On the other hand, medicine is facing a tremendous bureaucracy. When I finished my training, there was very little paperwork. Now, every action that is required to care for the patient has to be itemized and justified on paper. This incredible amount of paperwork is pure nonsense that has nothing to do with the practice of medicine and increases the cost of medical care. We are gradually being pushed from a profession into a business. We certainly need a tremendous overhaul of our health care system. I believe we need to keep medicine as a profession so that doctors don't start thinking of it as nine-to-five job. Physicians have always taken the responsibility for patients home with them. That is what has kept medicine a profession.

Medicine does require a lot of hours and hard work. I think that if you are happy in what you are doing, having to work more than eight hours a day becomes less important. Many physicians spend late nights taking care of patients or working on research projects in the lab. It became clear to me years ago that you don't have to be unusually smart to be a good doctor. You have to be willing to put in the extra time it takes to take care of people.

And common sense is essential. If you come across something you didn't expect to find and the result is for the better, don't pass it by. Think about why it turned out better. Take chance observations and use them for future opportunities.

Luck is when preparation meets with opportunity. I think the case of the woman from the watch factory is an example of that. An opportunity arose and I was fortunate to be in an institution that allowed me to investigate options to help her. Now she has helped us to help thousands of other people who need the same type of operation.

Stephen Ariyan is a former professor and chief of plastic surgery at Yale University School of Medicine. He is now an attending plastic surgeon at Yale.

6

At the End of the Line

 STAN THORNTON

Many of the cases I worked on my first year in practice were both legally and emotionally risky. As a resident, I decided to pursue my long-standing interest in children by concentrating in pediatric anesthesia. Soon after I was established in private practice in my hometown in Texas, I formed a relationship with a surgeon who also had an interest in pediatric cases. Working closely with him, I did anesthesia for the majority of pediatric cardiac cases at a major hospital in our area. These cases were challenging to me from a technical point of view, but they also have a high incidence of poor outcomes. The surgery can result in the death of the child or serious complications, such as stroke.

One of the cardiac patients I worked on with this surgeon was a three-year-old boy. He came to the hospital with an untreated infection, which had destroyed the main valve from his heart, the aortic valve. This leaky valve caused him to go into heart failure. I had the opportunity to anesthetize him several times for various interventions before we took him into the operating room. He was in the hospital for a total of six weeks before his surgery, so I got to know his family quite well.

The operation involved replacing the entire base of his aorta with a valve apparatus from a cadaver called an allograft. The surgical procedure was very risky, but it was the only hope that the child had. After making it through an eight- or nine-hour surgery, he died on the way to the intensive care unit. Facing this little boy's family was painful. I felt horrible. Everyone felt horrible. They had been prepared for this outcome. We told them from the beginning that the surgery was risky and there could be problems. Still, the last time they saw their three-year-old, he was smiling on the way into the operating room, and now he was gone.

It was easier for me to empathize with this family because I knew what they were going through. About a month after my wife and I moved to the area, our first child died of sudden infant death syndrome (SIDS). I know that there is absolutely nothing you can say to a family who loses a child. You can only tell them that you did all you could and try to reassure them that the baby didn't feel any pain. I don't tell people their child is in a better place now or that the angels have taken him, because I know I didn't want to hear anything like that. There are a lot more things *not* to say than there are things worth saying. You just have to let people grieve.

Now I find it's always more nerve-racking to do those types of cases. I'm sure my stress levels are high. I have had to learn to distance myself from it and not let it affect my judgment. If I ever stop and think about it, it always evokes those empty feelings I had when my baby died. I suppose this business I'm in, doing anesthesia for high-risk pediatric cases, is really setting me up to hurt more. But I know that I can do it well. Maybe in this way I can help prevent some families from having to experience the loss my wife and I did. And since I have this unique perspective, I can be more supportive to families when they do lose a loved one.

Coping with my child's death overshadowed many of my other concerns that year. Still, I also had a lot of anxiety about striking out on my own in a private practice. In residency, I always had an attending physician to fall back on during critical cases. But now I was completely responsible for everything that I did. There was no backup person to turn to for guidance—one of the most frightening things for me to get used to. This time, I was the end of the line. I am still not over that anxiety. My greatest fear going into practice was that I would be unable to be a competent practitioner. I even worried that I might kill my first few patients. Obviously, that did not turn out to be the case. As with any job, the more you do it the easier it gets. I probably did anesthesia for a thousand different surgeries that year. After the first few hundred, I was able to bolster my confidence.

Money was another source of anxiety for me when I first started my practice. I learned that when you begin billing, it takes three to six months to receive payments. I wasn't exactly sure how much I was going to make and if I was going to be able to pay my bills, but after the first few months I stopped worrying so much. I made more than enough money to cover my malpractice insurance premiums, put some money away for retirement, and pay for the house we bought. I was also able to retire all of my medical school debt rather quickly. Later, I found out it was unusual for a new physician to begin the way I did without joining another physician or a large group, although the start-up costs are less for anesthesia because we don't need any fancy office equipment. I guess I was lucky. Things fell into place financially for me very quickly.

In high school, I always liked science. I didn't know any physicians personally, but it seemed like that might be an interesting thing to do for a living. So, when I went to the University of Texas I majored in premed. I then went back home for four years of medical school. I spent four years in Pittsburgh, Pennsylvania, doing my anesthesiology residency. As a medical student, I thought about going into pediatrics or working in the intensive care unit. In the end, anesthesia, with its moment-to-moment decision making, appealed to me the most.

People often compare doing anesthesia to being a pilot—it's the takeoffs and landings that are critical. Also, you have to stay vigilant and monitor everything. If you make the wrong decision it can usually be pretty catastrophic. You have to have confidence in your decisions and act quickly. You also have to be somewhat like a pharmacist, keeping up with the literature on the latest drugs and understanding how they react with each other. Anesthesia is similar to surgery because it offers a lot of instant gratification. I like being able to give someone something and then see an immediate response.

Once I completed my residency and settled on a place to live, I had to decide what sort of practice I wanted. One option was to go into academics. As an academic anesthesiologist, at an institution where residents are being trained, you usually have a fairly reasonable schedule. You get several days off to prepare lectures and to teach. The hours aren't all that great, and in comparison to someone in private practice you do mostly supervisory work so you're not likely to be in the operating room 100 percent of the time. One advantage is that the university pays your salary, benefits, and malpractice premiums. If I decided to go into private practice, there were several settings to consider. I could choose to supervise one or two nurse anesthetists doing cases with me. It can be fairly lucrative, but you have to be legally responsible for a large number of cases and must always be available to respond to emergencies.

I chose a third option and set up a physician practice where I would do all the hands-on work and the mechanics of the surgery myself. As a self-employed physician, I have an office staff that does my billing and paperwork for me. I am personally responsible for keeping up-to-date my malpractice insurance, disability, and health and life insurance. I share an office with a group of other anesthesiologists, but we try to keep our professional affairs separate, mainly to avoid liability. If one person should be sued, the others would not be considered liable because they are not really partners, just co-owners of the office.

I had no real experience in my residency to compare with pure, physician-only, private-practice anesthesia. I tried to get a feel for what it would be like by visiting a couple of the anesthesiologists in the operating room and talking at length to seven or eight different physicians. I would recommend that someone who is looking to go into practice should try to get as much on-site information as possible. I had copies of the operating schedule for a week or so to get an idea of what sort of cases the anesthesiologists were doing. The first day I showed up at work, I had a full day's worth of cases and things have continued that way. I did not have to struggle to try to get to know surgeons and beg them for work—work was there for me automatically. My loose association with the anesthesiologists I shared an office with gave me a certain amount of credibility with the surgeons on staff, so I had an automatic referral base.

My typical daily routine was to wake up about 6:00 A.M. and get to the hospital usually by 7:00 A.M., where I would see the patients who were coming in that day for surgery. Our surgery schedule started at 8:00 A.M. For the majority of the day, I was in the operating room, aside from a few short trips to the recovery room to see patients who had surgery the day before. My day ended anywhere from 1:00 P.M. on a rather short day to 7:00 or

8:00 P.M. on a long day. The schedule was unpredictable on a day-to-day basis. Sometimes it was hard not knowing when I would be home on any given day, but unlike any of the other specialties, I often had afternoons off. Even though I couldn't plan anything, it still gave me a chance to spend some time with my family. In this practice, we were on call seven or eight times each month. That usually involved working until nine or ten at night. I got called out for a major surgery only 20 or 30 percent of the time.

Probably the most rewarding aspect of my first year was my affiliation with some of the surgeons who had an interest in pediatric cases. I was initially assigned to them by luck of the draw on the schedule. After watching me work, they began to ask for me again. When I realized that I had won the confidence of surgeons whom I respected, it was professionally very satisfying. I also began to be requested by individual patients, both adults and children. These were often friends or acquaintances of my family. Even more rewarding were the number of requests I had from patients who were co-workers at the hospital. These folks, being in a position to see my faults, still chose to place their trust in me to take care of them and their children. That also gave me more confidence in my abilities.

I did a lot of work with a urologic surgeon who specialized in spina bifida, a congential malformation of the lower portion of the spinal canal. People who have this disease are unable to empty their bladder sufficiently. It also causes lower extremity paralysis. The urologic management of this is rather complex. We would end up seeing the patients again and again. By the time these kids reach ten or twelve years old, they have had fifteen or twenty operations. The urologic reconstruction involved creating a bladder from stomach and/or intestine, which takes some time and is risky in some regards. We do these quite frequently, so we feel quite comfortable with them. The parents of these kids are usually very medically aware, but they require a lot of attention to help them through this stressful time. Usually the patients are very pleasant children who feel comfortable around health care workers and are a joy to work with.

These cases are not the rule, although they are the ones that had the most impact on me. I did do a lot of hysterectomies and tonsillectomies, but they were not as rewarding. There was also a twenty-year-old student at the hospital who took a bad fall and crushed his chest on a rock. He came in with an unstable broken neck and blood in his chest. The anesthesia for his treatment was very complicated. There were surgical and anesthetic complications every step of the way. Fortunately, everything went well. We didn't want the movement during chest surgery to disrupt his spinal cord, which was intact at the time, so I had to insert a breathing tube and turn him on his stomach, being careful not to disrupt his neck. After the surgeon fixed his neck, we turned him back over. I then woke him up to make sure he could still wiggle his toes and put him back to sleep for a chest procedure. Luckily, he didn't lose much blood or sustain any vascular injuries. The result was good. He did well, considering he had such a life-threatening injury.

Another patient was a friend of mine and my parents. He was a forty-year-old gentleman who had stomach ulcer symptoms and eventually succumbed to stomach cancer. I was able to take care of him for several of his surgeries. I helped serve as a liaison between his family and several of the other physicians who were taking care of him. This was another rewarding case because I knew I made a difference in the family's reaction to his health care even though the result was his death.

I do some personally challenging things in my practice and very risky things for some of the patients. Working with so many children and such high-risk surgeries, I expose myself to a lot of liability should there be an accident or an outcome that is less than favorable. I have been sued by the family of a child who had a complication after surgery; this was devastating to me but probably unavoidable. A lawyer told me physicians get sued an average of once every five years. I always heard that anesthesiologists, neurologists, and obstetricians get sued the most, but I never thought it would happen to me. This suit could be damaging to me financially and professionally if it is borne out. I hope it will be one of a very small number of suits that I'm involved in. It is already starting to wear on me—every time I get some correspondence from my lawyers, I get depressed about it. It makes you reevaluate everything you do. You feel like people automatically think you did the wrong thing.

I still take care of sick kids, but it has taken some work for me not to think about the lawsuit all the time. Should this malpractice lawsuit trend continue in the future, I will have to reduce the number of complex cases that I do now, unless someone else assumes the liability. It's just not worth it. In hindsight, I might have done better to choose a practice that allowed me to take care of mainly healthy patients at a surgery center or some smaller facility with less high-risk surgery. But then, I would not have experienced the many challenging and rewarding cases that I encountered my first year and continue to enjoy today.

Stan Thornton is an anesthesiologist in Texas.

7

Leading by Inspiration, Not by Fear

 THOMAS BREEN

Six months after I joined the faculty at the University of Massachusetts Medical School in Worcester as an orthopedic surgeon, I received a call from a medical center on the other side of the state, in Pittsfield. They wanted to refer a patient to us who was in a serious automobile accident earlier that week. The patient, a young man in his twenties, lost most of his elbow in the crash.

As the referring surgeon described the patient's condition, I thought of a case I worked on as an orthopedic surgery resident at Johns Hopkins in Baltimore. During my training with Dr. Andrew Weiland, a renowned hand surgeon, we performed a cadaveric elbow allograft transplant on a twenty-five-year-old man who lost his elbow in a motorcycle accident in Louisiana. I also wrote one of the few papers devoted to this unusual procedure during my hand surgery fellowship at Massachusetts General Hospital in Boston.

I felt this operation would be appropriate for the young man in Massachusetts because his original elbow joint was too damaged to salvage. A cadaveric elbow transplant had never been done before at U. Mass., but I thought it would be his only chance to keep a functioning arm. After the patient was transferred, we discussed the details of the procedure, and he was eager to proceed with it.

I found a suitable elbow joint from a bone bank in Florida, which sent us the frozen graft packed in dry ice. Operations of this magnitude need considerable preoperative planning. I outlined the surgical plan for the residents working under me, and we started at about 8:00 A.M. We were finished six hours later.

The operation involved inserting the cadaveric elbow into my patient's arm and attaching the graft to his own forearm and shoulder. We then reattached his muscles to the new elbow, allowing it to function again. He now has a useful range of motion in his elbow and works full-time as an operating room technician back in his hometown. Since that first operation, we have used this procedure many more times with good success.

The elbow transplant was the most vivid example of the way my mentors influenced me during my first year after my postgraduate training. The surgeons I trained under have served as excellent role models. When I became a faculty member, I tried to incorporate the best things they had to offer as I began training my own orthopedic surgery residents.

Many of the teaching techniques I used that first year were developed while I was a resident and fellow. While I was doing my hand surgery fellowship at Massachusetts General, we had weekly gross anatomy dissections. Each session was devoted to a different portion of the upper body that was dissected in minute detail and presented to the other residents and fellows under the critical eye of Drs. Richard Gelberman and Jesse Jupiter. I developed a keen interest in anatomy through these sessions. They showed me how essential anatomy is in surgery; it serves as the foundation of any operation. I adopted many of these anatomy teaching methods with my own residents and students.

The three surgeons I have mentioned as my role models were tough and demanding. They wanted things done right. They were fair, though, and just as hard on themselves as they were on us. They taught me how to organize a lecture that effectively drives home the important points. I also learned how to design a focused, concise research project.

I began to develop my own interpersonal style during my first year. I understood that the life of a resident can be very difficult, with long hours away from families and intense pressure to perform and succeed. Residents are usually in their late twenties or early thirties, but in medicine they are often treated like adolescents. I push my residents but make a conscious effort not to belittle or embarrass them in front of others. I have learned that you need to lead by inspiration, not by fear.

Teaching is a part of my academic position that I have always enjoyed. It forces me to keep up with current research and to contribute to my field. Part of my faculty position involved overseeing residents who were doing research. Orthopedics can be very mechanical. We are often dealing with screws, plates, stresses, and strains. There has been an explosion of different materials for prostheses and implants in the past twenty years. Many of my residents focused their studies in this area.

Whether I was in the laboratory or the operating room, there was always some form of teaching going on during my first year of practice. I never went through a day without having residents with me, discussing cases, basic concepts, and surgical techniques. I feel there is something to be gleaned from every case. We invest our medical skills in our patients, and they give so much in return, providing indispensable training for residents.

Since I had competed in sports in high school and college, I

always thought I would end up doing some sort of sports medicine. During my residency, however, I trained under one of the
world's great hand surgeons who inspired me to devote my career
to this subspecialty. I enjoy the intricate anatomy involved with
hand surgery and the fine detail of the procedures.

I had a chance to dovetail my interest in sports with my training
in hand surgery. About a month after I arrived in Worcester, we
operated on a professional baseball pitcher who had cut his hand
on a piece of glass. He had cut many tendons and nerves, so
the injury was potentially devastating to his career. The accident
happened during the off-season, and he wanted to be able to play
the following spring. He had a good recovery and went on to have
a successful season pitching in the major leagues.

As a fellow at Massachusetts General, I had many opportunities
to become involved in treating professional athletes. It was gratifying to treat them because they are motivated to recover and return
to the playing field. Cases like the professional pitcher and the
elbow transplant gave me a challenging start in my career.

That first year, my schedule was full and diverse. I split my
time between teaching, research, and seeing patients in the clinic
and the operating room. The actual hours that I worked were
a little better than residency. But since there is more emotional
investment when you are the attending surgeon, I felt as if I was
working harder. Suddenly, I was the one that everybody was looking to for answers.

On a typical day, I got to my office at the medical school by
6:30 A.M. to make rounds before the 7:00 A.M. resident teaching
conference. I used the Socratic method during the conference to
teach residents about specific cases or clinical problems. After the
conference ended at 7:30 A.M., I would either see patients in the
clinic or go directly into surgery. I operated two full days a week
my first year—one day in outpatient surgery and one day in in-

patient. There was not a day that went by when I did not bring work home with me that was impossible to finish during the day.

In addition to beginning a new career, I also got married my first year in practice. My wife, Susan, and I got married after she finished her residency in New York six months after I came to Worcester. She is an ophthalmologist. When Susan and I started our lives together, it was quite an adjustment to learn to think "we" and not "me."

It is easy to get consumed by all these adjustments. Many new things were happening to us all at once. To relieve stress, I spent many hours bicycle racing on spring and summer weekends. I also rode my bike to work many days, which gave me time to think and get workouts during otherwise full weeks. Being involved in athletics helped me keep a balanced outlook. I developed a lot of nonmedical friends that year, which also helped me keep my career in perspective.

Every now and then, Susan and I would take off to Boston or Vermont for the weekend. But our first year was so consuming, we did not do this as much as we would have liked. Going through a common experience helped us support each other and definitely made our first year in practice more tolerable and enjoyable.

During my first year, I learned that there are many things about going into practice that they just don't teach you in medical school. It is a rude awakening when you find out that medicine also involves an immense bureaucracy. When you come out of your residency or fellowship, you are all geared up to treat patients and contribute to your field when you realize you are getting bombarded with extraneous duties. Hospital politics, workers' compensation, and malpractice insurance can be frustrating to deal with when they cut into your hectic workdays. The steady stream of paperwork encroaches upon your practice and, at times, takes some of the fun out of it.

I also found out that patients who have surgery do not always return to normal, which is a hard thing to accept when you invest so much energy trying to make them better. When you decide to perform an operation, you are putting something of yourself on the line. If the result is less than optimal, you tend to take it personally.

Sometimes I ran into patients who were angry or suspicious. The threat of being sued is pervasive in medicine. Physicians tend to be defensive and hedge their bets. You tend to order more tests and X rays to be absolutely sure. This atmosphere has disillusioned many physicians and caused some to drop out of medicine. Today, there are many courses physicians can take to learn how to improve patient care and minimize practice behaviors that leave them vulnerable to being sued. I feel it would be helpful if there were more emphasis placed on better doctor/patient communication and on record keeping during residency. It would be money well spent for residents to get involved in this before starting their own practice.

Because I specialized in hand surgery, I saw a large number of patients who were injured at work. Many of the injuries were devastating and called for immediate surgery. If someone got a hand crushed in a machine, for example, that was a very obvious problem that I could treat in a concrete way. Other patients who came in for treatment did not have any visible abnormality. These vague complaints were more difficult to diagnose and treat because I could not document them with objective tests. The workers' compensation patients, as a group, generally have poorer results because they are not motivated to get better, which was very frustrating because I put a lot of time into treating them. During residency, you think all patients want to get better. Working with this group of workers' compensation patients was another difficult and unexpected adjustment my first year in practice.

The most fulfilling part of my workday was the time I spent teaching residents. Medicine is an apprenticeship, and I enjoyed passing along the knowledge my mentors gave me to the next generation of physicians. Since that first elbow transplant I performed, I have done many similar operations. I find them to be an excellent teaching technique for residents. Some of the men and women I have trained have gone on to do a hand surgery fellowship and perform the same type of operation in hospitals where they set up practice.

Generally, people in academic medicine make less than people in private practice, but being in academics keeps me up-to-date and gives me a chance to contribute something new to my specialty. Working with residents is very satisfying; I push them hard and they challenge me right back.

Thomas Breen is an assistant professor in the department of orthopedics at the University of Massachusetts in Worcester, Massachusetts. He specializes in hand surgery.

8

Mr. Jenkins's Holy Ghost

 J. MEADOR-WOODRUFF

The pager woke me from a restless sleep. It was the resident summoning me to join her in the emergency room. Wearing a beeper was a new experience for me: I was a third-year medical student starting my psychiatry rotation, and this was my first night on call.

I had just completed three months of internal medicine and was considering a career in gastroenterology. As an undergraduate, I studied intestinal enzymes in a biochemistry laboratory, so that seemed to be the way to go at the time. The problem was, I did not enjoy my internal medicine rotation. I was at a loss as to what other specialty I might find interesting, so I decided to keep an open mind about psychiatry.

Wondering what kind of psychiatric problem would cause someone to end up in the emergency room at three in the morning, I climbed out of bed and found the ER.

The resident was waiting for me when I got there. She said the patient, Mr. Jenkins, was a schizophrenic who was well known to all of the house staff. He was middle aged and periodically came in when he went off his antipsychotic medications. His usual pattern was that he would decide he no longer needed his medicine, and about ten days later come into the ER hearing voices telling him to kill himself.

I had never seen a schizophrenic patient in the flesh. I studied the textbook enough to know that schizophrenia is not a state of having multiple personalities, a view that has somehow found its way into the public's perception of this illness. I also knew it was a progressive psychotic disorder, which causes patients to experience hallucinations and delusions. Schizophrenics are often unable to work, maintain normal relationships, or take care of their basic needs.

The resident and I stepped into Mr. Jenkins's room. The chart indicated that he was about forty, but he looked considerably older. He had not bathed in days, and his clothes were dirty and disheveled. He was pacing around the room talking to himself.

After we introduced ourselves, the patient settled down a bit but was too restless to sit down for long. I do not remember the specifics of the interview years later, but I was struck by one aspect of it: Mr. Jenkins introduced me to his "holy ghost." This patient could both see and hear another individual in the room with us, whom he called his holy ghost. He said his holy ghost was benevolent and was often with him, providing a running verbal commentary about what he was doing, thinking, and feeling at any given moment.

When we entered the room, Mr. Jenkins said he had not been talking to himself but to this entity. We hospitalized him and he partially responded to treatment.

This was the first psychotic individual I had ever talked to, and it made a significant impression on me. I became convinced that this man really did see and hear someone whom I could not perceive. I did not understand how this could happen and soon discovered that no one else—including members of the psychiatry department—could explain the phenomenon of psychosis. It seemed that something was fundamentally wrong with the way the nervous system was wired in these individuals, but the secret was not revealed to me that year.

I was able to see more schizophrenics and other mentally ill patients as I completed my psychiatry rotation. When I went on to my other third-year rotations, my mind kept coming back to the man in the ER who had his holy ghost with him. I wondered what could be causing his bizarre behavior and sensory experiences. At the end of the year, I arranged an elective rotation in the psychiatry department to learn more about schizophrenia.

The first patient I saw on that rotation was a chronic paranoid schizophrenic named Mr. Meyer, who was also well known to the residents. He was admitted to my service shortly after pulling his right eyeball out.

Many schizophrenic patients have delusions and hallucinations with a religious theme. They believe they are deities, that they have some direct access to God, or that they can hear the voice of God. A smaller group of schizophrenics report hearing a voice, often attributed to God, quoting a biblical verse: "If thy evil eye offend thee, pluck it out." Mr. Meyer heard the voice commanding him to do this, and he acted on it. Sadly, he had heard the same voice five years before and had gouged out his left eye, so he was now totally blind. We were able to help him feel less agitated after a few weeks of treatment, but his psychosis was severe and barely controlled.

I took care of another schizophrenic patient later that week who had elements of catatonia, an unusual set of symptoms that involves the motor system. This patient, Mr. Fraser, stood in bizarre postures for hours at a time, with little or no voluntary movement. He would often strike a pose standing in front of a window with his arms curled above his head. He resisted any efforts to put his arms at his side.

Perhaps due to my naivete, I asked him why he was doing this. Mr. Fraser attempted to explain in disjointed sentences. I learned that he thought he was a tree, and his outspread arms were his branches. By standing in front of the window, he was trying to obtain enough sunlight to provide nutrition for his body through photosynthesis.

These schizophrenic patients intrigued me, so after much deliberation, I decided to pursue a career in psychiatry. I had entered medicine to help people in need, and I could find no group of patients in more need of compassionate care than these profoundly psychotic individuals. So much was known about the cause of many other medical problems, but it seemed to me that little of substance was known about the causes of major mental illness.

Early in my postgraduate training, I discovered a much darker side to schizophrenia. Before, I had been exposed only to the so-called positive symptoms, the dramatic hallucinations and delusions. As my sophistication grew, I became more aware of the negative symptoms of the illness. These pervasive symptoms include lack of energy, flat affect, depression, apathy, and the inability to experience pleasure or interact appropriately with people. These negative symptoms, along with the hallucinations and delusions, contributed to the poor social functioning of almost all of the schizophrenic patients.

Most of my patients were unemployed, often homeless and living from shelter to shelter. They were unable to sustain any sort of interpersonal relationship and often attempted to medicate themselves with alcohol and a variety of other drugs. I found that a large percentage of the homeless are mentally ill. They are not destitute by choice.

Antipsychotic medications helped the patients cope with the

more florid symptoms such as hallucinations, but they did not diminish the negative symptoms much or help correct their bleak social situations. A large number of patients develop a serious side effect after many years of treatment that causes uncontrollable, abnormal body movements. This phenomenon, called tardive dyskinesia, may occur in up to a quarter of all patients treated with the antipsychotics for a long period of time.

Not all schizophrenics are this impaired. But since I did my residency in a large and well-known program at the University of Michigan, I saw many patients who were referred by community psychiatrists. These physicians often refer their most difficult cases to university hospitals for evaluation and treatment, especially when the limited available treatments fail to help.

I was also fortunate to see some schizophrenics who did fairly well. One patient I saw throughout my residency was able to hold a well-paying technical job and was married to a very informed, supportive spouse. This patient, Mr. Griffin, became psychotic about once a year, usually in the late fall or early winter. We identified this trend together.

He was able to recognize certain symptoms that warned him of an impending psychosis. He learned to ward it off by adjusting his medication dose when the red-flag symptoms occurred. Mr. Griffin has managed to stay out of the hospital for years and has done reasonably well. Unfortunately, many schizophrenics do not do nearly so well.

It was clear to me that something was fundamentally wrong with the way the brain of a schizophrenic works. I knew that it probably involved a subtle imbalance in the brain that leads to profound behavioral symptoms. Early in my training, I reached an additional decision point that has shaped my career to date. I asked myself "In what setting could I deal most effectively with this illness?"

On the one hand I could be a clinician who treats these patients in a traditional practice setting. I could also go into research to try to understand the cause of schizophrenia and develop better treatments. At the time, I felt the available treatments were only marginally effective. I decided that I would be most effective in a research setting and embarked on an extensive training period to prepare for a career in this arena.

During the beginning of my training, I learned a number of techniques that would help me perform research in schizophrenia. While I had performed research both as an undergraduate and as a medical student, there were many additional skills that I had to master to be able to do the types of studies I envisioned. Since schizophrenia is likely a disease of chemical transmission in the brain, I decided to undertake a direct study of the schizophrenic brain.

A number of methods are available to study the brain, but they all have significant limitations. One method that has recently gained popularity is to study a living person's brain by using radiological techniques such as positron emission tomography, or PET scans. Due to the limits of the technique, however, only relatively large areas of the brain can be seen. To study schizophrenia, researchers need to focus on smaller cellular details.

I decided to study directly the brains of schizophrenic patients who have died. This method has the advantage of providing minute levels of resolution and the potential to yield exciting data about the underlying chemical defects in this illness. But it can be difficult to obtain sufficient numbers of brains to study.

The first step in such an endeavor is to find a source of brains. As part of a larger research group, I identified a hospital in my area known to have many aging schizophrenics who had been chronically institutionalized. By approaching the hospital, patients, and their families, we were able to set up a donation network for a brain bank.

Setting up the donation program was a time-consuming process. Brains have to be removed quickly during an autopsy and prepared for later study. Once a patient has died and the family agrees to donate his or her brain, the hospital records have to be examined carefully. We also interviewed the hospital staff and the family to verify the psychiatric diagnosis. Unfortunately, many patients have been diagnosed with schizophrenia but do not actually have the illness when a careful diagnostic assessment is undertaken.

Once the brain is collected and the patient is clinically assessed, the brain is prepared for storage. Part of it is frozen and the rest is fixed in formaldehyde. I have been able to acquire about one brain a month.

After I found a supply of brains, I had to decide which chemicals in the brain to study. There are literally hundreds if not thousands of chemicals in the brain that could be involved in schizophrenia, or for that matter in any aspect of brain functioning. Fortunately, in the 1960s and 1970s, it became clear that the medications we use to treat schizophrenia all have the ability to block the actions of the brain chemical dopamine.

Dopamine is a neurotransmitter, or brain chemical, that is known to be involved in regulating emotions and controlling the motor system. Because antipsychotic medications tend to block the effects of dopamine at its specific receptors in the brain, this suggests that schizophrenia may be associated with a relative abundance of dopamine in the brain. Despite extensive prior study, however, the exact nature of this presumed dopamine excess has not been established.

During my first year of training in this area of psychiatry, an exciting discovery was made in dopamine neurochemistry. The gene that is responsible for the synthesis of a dopamine receptor (a molecule on the outside of a cell that interacts with dopamine) was identified and cloned. Shortly thereafter, four additional genes were discovered that also code for other dopamine receptors. This was unexpected. Two dopamine receptors had previously been suspected, but the discovery of five different genes led to a number of possibilities in terms of how dopamine functions in the brain, and may be disturbed in schizophrenia.

Although we are still in a very early stage in this field of investigation, a number of interesting and exciting discoveries have already been made that it is hoped will explain how these chemical disturbances become disordered in psychosis.

Despite the rapid progress and exciting findings in this field, the actual laboratory setting used by researchers tends to be quite modest. It only takes a few small rooms to do all of the studies on the brains themselves.

Selected regions of the brains are removed from the freezer and mounted onto small steel blocks. They are then cut into paper-thin slices and mounted on large glass microscope slides. After the tissue slices are treated with a series of chemicals, radioactive markers that chemically bind to dopamine receptors or their gene products are applied. When the slide is exposed to an X-ray film or photographic emulsion, an image appears that shows exactly where these molecules occur in the brain and just how much is present in any given cell.

The technique helps researchers decipher how these chemical systems operate in the brain. By studying the differences between a normal brain and a schizophrenic brain, we can begin to understand how these systems are disordered in the illness.

My primary effort today continues to be performing basic laboratory research into fundamental questions of how regions of the brain are connected, how dopamine and other chemicals are involved in those connections, and how these symptoms function in the brains of schizophrenics.

Many exciting developments have occurred in this field since I began, and some hold considerable promise for the development of more effective and safer treatments for schizophrenia. But I have never forgotten that first patient, Mr. Jenkins, and his holy ghost. To avoid losing sight of my goal of helping these individuals, I continue to see a number of schizophrenic patients in my clinic, helping them to deal with the daily problems of living with a chronic mental illness.

James Meador-Woodruff studies schizophrenia at the University of Michigan's Mental Health Research Institute in Ann Arbor, Michigan.

9

Making the Switch to Pharmaceuticals

 DEBRA WILLIAMS

Before I became a pharmaceutical researcher, I was on the faculty at an East Coast medical school. I spent part of my time in the intensive care unit (ICU) as an attending physician. On top of that, I had several basic science research projects going. I served on a couple of committees, and put in a few hours a week at an outside clinic. I enjoyed my work, and if I didn't have any outside life, it would have been fine, but I have two little boys. I found out it was impossible to do all those things and still have a family life.

For a working mother, I had the best of all possible worlds. I had a full-time nanny living in, so I could leave the house at five in the morning if I wanted to and somebody would be taking care of the kids. My husband did all the cooking. Somebody came in to do the cleaning. I had the maximum support system, yet it was still impossible. The bottom line is the kids never saw me. I came to the pharmaceutical firm more for the sake of family harmony than anything else. My husband, who has worked there in the basic science division for thirteen years, got frustrated with my heavy schedule. He encouraged me to give them a copy of my CV. A few days later, they called me for an interview. I wasn't very interested and I had no experience in running clinical trials, but I went anyway to be a good sport. At that point, I wasn't ready to leave academics yet.

After another month in the ICU, I was completely burned out. Direct patient care gets so draining after a while, especially hospital care. The pressure is so intense and constant. You do a little good for some of the people, but for a lot of them, you don't do anything. I started to reach a point where it was not interesting or challenging anymore. It's rewarding when you see people get better, but when it becomes rote, the interest is gone. I finally called the pharmaceutical firm. They were still interested, so I took the job. I really had no idea what I was getting into, but I've been happy ever since. There are some very bright people here.

Since my background is in research—I got a Ph.D. in immunology before I went to medical school—I always thought I would end up in research, but not in the pharmaceutical industry. I don't believe anybody in medicine considers that directly. If they know anything about it, they think it's sort of a dead-end job for retired doctors or somebody who can't make it in practice or something. Times are changing. It used to be harder to get young people right out of training into the pharmaceutical industry. When we have a position open now, we're getting some really good CVs in. Too few medical students consider this option. For me, it was a very rewarding career choice that fit well with my family's needs.

During my first year in pharmaceutical research, I was amazed by the difference in working environments. I couldn't plan my life when I was at the ICU because I never knew when I would be put on call for a holiday.

The situation in my research position was much better. Suddenly I had the freedom to plan vacations when I wanted and to be home at a reasonable time most nights. Physicians are happy coming into the pharmaceutical industry because the fifty- or sixty-hour weeks they're comfortable working are considered long hard hours to everybody else. From the very beginning people thought I was doing a good job, and I got promoted after two years. It's a much more positive system of rewards. A lot of people came here making a lifestyle decision, so it's a much more family-oriented environment. Nobody would give it a second thought if my kids were sick and I had to leave early. My boss would be kicking me out of here, saying, "Go home for your kids." This place is cleared out generally at six o'clock. On weekends, people are not expected to come in. (There were rare times when everyone came in on weekends to work on special projects.) Another nice thing about coming here was that the hassle factor was gone. I had a secretary who took care of arranging travel; if I had to go to a meeting somewhere, she would organize it. I didn't have to take care of photocopying; somebody would do it for me. Finally, I had more time to really use my mind instead of devoting my energy to scheduling conflicts and clerical things.

During my first year here, I helped set up a compassionate program that provided free experimental drugs for AIDS treatment. One of the antibiotics developed for routine sore throats and pneumonia also had activity against some of the bacterial and parasitic infections that AIDS patients get. Two of those infections had no prior drugs to treat them. Some pilot studies were just starting, but we also opened these compassionate programs for people who couldn't tolerate conventional therapy if there was any, or whose conventional treatment was failing.

One of my most gratifying experiences was working with patients and their families to help them get started on the drug. The program was still in the design phase when a mother telephoned my office. She asked me, "Do you prohibit children in your studies?"

I said, "Of course not."

She asked, "Do they have to have AIDS?"

"Of course not," I said.

She suddenly burst into tears on the other end of the phone. "Oh thank God," she said. "This was my last hope for my son."

The woman's child had an unusual underlying immunodeficiency that gave him the same sort of infections that AIDS patients get. She had apparently called another company with more strict criteria that wouldn't give the drug out for kids and made it available only to AIDS patients.

"My son is very sick, how soon can we get it?" she asked.

"We haven't got the program started for this drug yet," I said, "but if his physician feels he needs it, we'll call and get approval."

After speaking with his physician, we called the FDA that day and got permission. We got the drug out to their physician within a week. Later on, the child couldn't take oral drugs, so he had to take it intravenously. He was the first person in the United States to use the intravenous form. We got that to him on Thanksgiving Day. His mother was so grateful. Two years later, the child is doing very well.

A while later, a physician called my office about a ten-year-old girl who got AIDS from a transfusion.

"She's in the hospital burning up with a 107-degree temperature," he said. "We have no other drugs to treat her with. I was wondering if we could get some of this new drug for her."

"Yes," I said. "We can certainly make it available to you." We got the drug out to him the next day. Five days later, he reported that the girl's fever was gone. Ten days later, she left the hospital. Her mother was ready to testify in front of Congress because it was the best quality of life her daugher has had after trying AZT, ddi, and many other drugs.

Some of the saddest calls came from AIDS patients who were resistant to drugs that were similar to ours. They would call to try to get our drug and we would tell them, "Because you're resistant to the other drug, you will also be resistant to our drug. It won't work for you." We felt as if we were giving them a death sentence. But through the physicians we also heard a lot of stories about people who were doing well. These compassionate programs took a lot of time outside of my regular duties that year, but they were very satisfying. They were a lot of work for the secretaries and the people who kept track of all the data, but we all put our hearts and souls into it because we knew how important it was.

Like many people, I used to think that physicians in the pharmaceutical industry had very little contact with patients. But I interacted with many patients and their loved ones through this compassionate program. We sometimes knew more about these kids than their physicians did. By tracking all their paperwork over time and corresponding with their physicians, we became very attached to the patients in the program.

In the beginning, I wasn't thrown into anything very complicated. I was hired to be responsible for developing asthma drugs. The drugs had passed safety testing in phase one trials, where a drug that has been cleared in animals goes into young male volunteers to make sure it is safe for humans. Next, there might be a couple of phase two pilot studies to see if the drug works for asthma patients. Then it goes into phase three, which includes all the studies necessary to get the drug approved by the FDA. I was hired to organize the phase two and phase three studies on these drugs.

During that first year, I was part of a team that was deciding whether these compounds could safely be tested on people. The minute a new compound is identified, a new team is formed with somebody from the science group, the toxicology group, and the chemistry group, who would get together frequently to make all the decisions about what to do with the drug. Early on, one drug looked very promising, but it caused an unusual toxicity. It was something that couldn't be picked up by any early test, and the end result was a permanent change. I said, "There's no way I'll test this compound on a human being." Everybody turned around and said, "Well, I guess you're right about that." I made the recommendation that we drop the compound, and the committee approved it. When a clinician is seriously challenging safety, usually everybody goes with the more conservative view.

It was a new experience for me to be in a position where people listened to what I had to say and took it seriously. It was a whole new environment, working on a team. Everybody's opinion in their area of expertise is considered important. Here, you have to work for the good of the company. The kind of physician who won't do well in the pharmaceutical industry is someone who enjoys being in charge and giving orders to the nurses. There's no place for that here.

I was an associate director my first year in research. That's the entry-level title for a physician in the pharmaceutical industry. I used to spend the first hour of the morning in the library going through all the journals to see if there were any new studies related to asthma or whatever else I was working on. Then I usually returned phone calls to physicians who wanted to enroll their patients in the compassionate program or wanted information about the drug. There would usually be two or three meetings a day of a half hour to an hour each. It might be the lab meeting with the basic science group, the asthma team, or with the other people in the compassionate program. Next, I might have made a presentation to some management committee, updating them on the status of clinical studies and our plan for the asthma drugs. I also spent about an hour each day sitting down with the clinical research associates who do all the actual work for the studies in the field. We would talk about how best to set up a new study or how they planned to travel to the various sites where the drug would be distributed.

Designing, running, and analyzing clinical studies is a long process that usually takes eighteen months. First, you research the literature to find out what is the best way to run an asthma study, then you design it and write the protocol. You work with the clinical research associates on how to implement it to make it run smoothly. Then you identify all the people who might be interested in doing the study. We usually recruit these people from academics. They might be in asthma centers or clinics that can provide enough patients for what we're doing. We talk to the investigators, we go out and visit all those sites to make sure they have a good clinic, a pharmacy, and a lab. We do a background check to make sure they've never committed fraud or anything illegal. We call up the pharmacy and order as much of the drug as we need for the trials. I would also talk to the statistician about the size of study I would need. For the big studies that we submit to the FDA for approval, there are often three hundred patient studies at forty centers around the country.

At some point, we would have all the various people doing the studies get together in what is called an investigator's meeting. Then, the associates go out to start up the sites, to tell them which blood tests we need drawn each month, and to show them how the forms need to be filled out and what safety precautions they have to take. During the study, if there are any medical or safety questions that come up, the people call us. I would be the person to take care of any medical problems that came up along the way. Once all the data are in, the analysis starts. We write the study reports, which are filed with the FDA. I might also work with some of the investigators to write a publication about it.

That's the baseline job of somebody in the pharmaceutical industry—to design, run, and analyze studies and to monitor safety problems. Meanwhile, I also kept my own clinic. The firm I work for allows all physicians to practice one-half day a week, so on Wednesday mornings I was seeing pulmonary patients over at the veteran's hospital where I had my clinic. I've got patients I've been taking care of for seven years now, so I've still got that continuity of care. A lot of the lung disease I see in the veterans is related to asthma or is treated similarly, so that fits in with what I'm doing here. I don't feel I'm out of touch with medicine. In fact I've learned a lot of medicine working with pharmaceuticals.

It's too bad that most medical school graduates don't consider this type of job in pharmaceuticals as a worthwhile career. Part of that is a bias on the part of physicians who have never been exposed to the pharmaceutical industry. If you're around physicians who have never been involved in clinical trials, the one interaction they have with the pharmaceutical industry is with sales representatives. What may be a negative feeling about sales representatives carries over to the industry in general. It's changing, though. I know several people who have gone on to work in the pharmaceutical industry and they all are very happy about it. The word is getting around about all these talented people who walked away from academic medicine.

Pharmaceutical companies don't want students right out of medical school; you need some sort of training. It could be internal medicine or a fellowship in pulmonary medicine, cardiology, or clinical pharmacology. These are areas with major sections of drugs. Other up-and-coming areas to specialize in are immunology and biotechnology. A Ph.D. or some good basic science training in molecular biology or immunology would also be good. What they want is somebody who knows the language and who has a good feel for what is going on in medicine as well as in research.

Although I ended up in pharmaceutical research somewhat by accident, I feel it is an excellent fit for me. I never wanted to be a full-time doctor. I grew up in a rural area; I knew how hard general practitioners worked and I wanted no part of that lifestyle. I wanted to be able to have a family and a life of my own outside of work. I found out I couldn't do it in academic medicine, either. In research, I have found the perfect balance of intellectual challenge and patient contact, with enough time left over for a happy family life.

Debra Williams is a clinical researcher at a pharmaceutical firm in Connecticut.

10

Memoir of a Forensic Pathologist

 WERNER SPITZ

In the seven years that I worked as a pathologist in Jerusalem, I saw only one murder. You don't go into this profession to avoid seeing violent death, so I decided to go to the United States so I could see more cases. I went through New York to get to Baltimore, where I had found a job in the medical examiner's office. I arrived on a Saturday evening. When I came to New York, they told me the next plane to Baltimore was in eight hours, so I sat and waited. I went to a restaurant, but I didn't understand the menu, so I said to the girl behind the counter, "Give me the same as he has," pointing to the guy next to me.

When I finally got to Baltimore, I hailed a cab. I told the driver to take me to the medical examiner's office. "Oh," he said. "You mean the morgue." He drove me to the waterfront in a miserable part of town. I looked out and saw a ramshackle building and said, "This can't be it." I went to the front door and walked up a set of steel steps. Through a window, I saw fifteen open bodies. I said to myself, "Well, this must be it after all."

It was July 1 when I arrived. The temperature was 106 degrees in Baltimore, and I was dressed in a woollen jacket that was more suited for the middle of winter. As I stood there looking at the bodies, my new boss came up to me and said, "You must be Dr. Spitz." He lent me a beat-up old Cadillac, and I went that day to look for a place to live. I ended up sharing a place around the corner from the morgue with one of the residents.

The building was terrible and the equipment was miserable. Much of it was homemade by the doctors, but I learned a whole lot and the people I worked with were wonderful. I had fifteen open bodies every day in Baltimore. We had about four hundred to five hundred murder cases in one year. That was a lot better than the one case I had in Israel in seven years. I never in my remotest dreams thought I would be exposed to such an overwhelming amount of material.

On a typical day, I got to work at 8:30 A.M. I was allocated a number of cases, which were usually either murders, suicides, or accidental deaths. In the morning I worked with the police to get information, made phone calls, did autopsies, and made reports. In any autopsy, you look for anything that shows up that is not normal. That's the last opportunity you have to get certain details. You always collect tissues for microscope work and lab work. You collect blood, urine, and sometimes eye fluid or spinal fluid. In the afternoon, I was often called to testify in court on the various cases. After grabbing a quick bite, I would go back to the office and work into the evening on experiments. Every third week, I would work seven days in a row because I was on call for the weekend. I had no money for a telephone, so I used to run around the corner every half hour until midnight to see if they needed me for anything.

I was the new kid on the block with all these other residents. We weren't pushed to excel, but everybody tried to do better than anybody else. Some didn't dream of investing an extra hour in work that was not directly expected of them in their contract, but I was devoting a lot of time to work outside what was required. Most of the time, when other people went out on the town, I was in the back room of the morgue. My wife, who I was dating at that time, used to come help me. Afterward we might go out for a hamburger. That would be our evening. Many people would say, "I don't want to invest my young years in that kind of nonsense," and I don't blame them. But there is absolutely no doubt that if I didn't do all those things, I wouldn't be where I am today.

I was working on drowning experiments at the time. It never seemed logical to me that people could drown of asphyxiation. Merely having water in the lungs does not cause death. I published a study on this topic based on experiments I did at the morgue. Those experiments paid off for me. When they wanted an autopsy of Mary Jo Kopechne, the girl who went over the bridge in Chappaquiddick, I got the case because of my expertise in causes of death by drowning. People who die in fresh water or brackish water with a low salinity draw the water into their blood through the lungs. The blood becomes diluted with all the low salt water that comes in. This overburdens the heart, dilutes all the chemicals in the blood, and causes the blood cells to break up. The police thought she might have been dead before she went down, but I testified that she was alive. By looking at pictures that were taken before she was buried, I saw foam in her airways, which showed that she was breathing at the time.

Originally, when the girl died, the authorities decided they would not do an autopsy. But three months later, after there was so much publicity, the attorney general from Massachusetts tried to get her body exhumed to find out if she was pregnant. Her family was opposed to the idea. I testified in court that an autopsy after burial would not yield anything. An autopsy should have been done three months earlier. The case was tried in Pennsylvania. I remember arriving back in the Baltimore airport and seeing my picture on page one of all the newspapers. I guess I was probably impressed with myself.

That was one of the cases that gave me a national reputation. I also testified in the assassination of John F. Kennedy. They were trying to determine whether there was reason to believe there was a conspiracy. If he was shot from the front and the back, that would mean there were two people. I reviewed the autopsy materials that had accumulated for the case. I found, with absolutely no question, that he was not shot from two sides. More recently, I have given expert testimony in the "preppie murder case" and some of the Kevorkian suicides. Most of my forty years in medicine were spent in Detroit, as the Wayne County coroner.

If you want to be someone, you have to publish. I publish my work at every opportunity. Today, after forty years in the profession, I have published eighty-nine papers and a textbook. You don't become known around the world by just doing good work. Just getting a good job and doing an eight- or ten-hour day is not enough. We are as good as our peers think we are. When we've gotten to the point where our peers look up to us, or even think of us as an equal, then we have made it. That's what we have to strive for. You have to make the time, because you don't need to sleep eight hours. You have to do it when you are young and eager and energetic. Still, it's not an easy specialty to go into.

Pathology is grisly. It's bloody and gory and messy, but you don't really see the gore and smell the nasty odor because it's a job. Somehow, your brain shifts gears. You don't experience all the nastiness because you do it day in and day out. If you don't think about what led up to a death, it becomes a thing, not a person anymore. I went to see the movie *Jaws* a few years ago. During the part when the shark bit the girl's leg and there was blood all over, I walked out. I knew it was only a movie, but I couldn't stand the pain and suffering. In 1987 I was called to a plane crash at Detroit Metro Airport, where 156 people died. Family members came to ask me if their friends or relatives were on the plane. They cried and I wanted to cry with them, but I couldn't show my emotions. When I started to feel bad, I walked back to where the bodies were. I felt better in there because I didn't see them as people who were suffering. Maybe that shows I wouldn't have been a terribly good clinician.

When I was growing up, there was never a question in my family about whether I would go to medical school. My father was an internist, and I wanted to be a physician, too. The same thing happened with my son. I asked him what he was going to do after college and he said, "Well, what else is there?" My interest in pathology began when I was in medical school in Jerusalem. My father didn't want me to be home doing nothing for three months during summer vacation, so he got me a job as a "gofer" in the pathology department at the city hospital, where I would be exposed to something medical. If the floor in the autopsy room had blood on it, I washed it. Gradually, they gave me more responsibility. The third summer I spent there, they let me do an autopsy. I had already watched several hundred by that time. Apparently, I did it quite well. The autopsy took me seven hours, and I was completely exhausted. Today, I do it in twenty-five minutes. When it came time to pick a residency, I couldn't make up my mind. I decided, "Well, since I know pathology a little bit, why don't I start with pathology and maybe change my mind later." A month, then six weeks went by, and I still hadn't made up my mind. I was getting more responsibility demonstrating autopsies for clinicians. Six more weeks went by. I decided, "Well, maybe I'll try six more weeks of pathology." The six weeks became the rest of my life.

When you choose a career, you have to be pretty careful about what you do because changing directions is difficult, especially in medicine. I don't think medical students give pathology enough consideration. People want to go into specialties where they can help patients rather than doing so after the fact. A person who goes into pathology should at least be attracted by the desire to be helpful in educating clinicians about the processes of disease found in an autopsy. There are a lot of avenues for research. A person who goes into pathology should understand that it is different from having direct contact with patients. A pathologist is more or less a laboratory person who helps determine the causes of disease. In that way, the specialty provides an opportunity to help people now, and into the future.

Werner Spitz, now semiretired, is the former coroner in Wayne County, Michigan.

11

Medicine and Motherhood

 MARY ALFANO

A woman's voice came over the hospital loudspeaker and interrupted my lunch to announce an urgent case in the emergency room. As one of the residents on staff, I was supposed to come running whenever that happened. But this time, there was a slight problem. I was very pregnant with my ten-pound son, and he was due any day. I remember inserting an endotracheal tube to help this patient breathe, hoping nothing would happen because I was having contractions every three minutes.

Since I had my son, Zachary, two days after my residency ended, I spent my first year in practice nursing a newborn and going without sleep many nights when he was sick or decided to wait up for me and visit during the night. I took a position with a university student clinic ten weeks after I finished my residency. I was biding time, waiting for a faculty position to open up at the medical school there. At the clinic, I had stable hours, 8:30 A.M. to 5:00 P.M., five days a week, and no nights on call. I wanted something that would give me easier hours with my baby, and it fit the bill.

Being pregnant during my residency and nursing my son during my first couple of years in practice presented a challenge, but it was not the first time I had to overcome obstacles on my path to becoming a doctor. My year at the clinic working with young college students confirmed for me that I wanted to go into primary care. It also showed me that I wanted to take care of patients with a broader range of ages and medical problems, as I had in my family practice residency.

I saw between thirty and fifty patients a day in the outpatient clinic. The students were mostly from middle- and upper-class families. They were all between eighteen and twenty-five, with ailments such as asthma attacks, sexually transmitted diseases, and depression. Some patients I might see for only ten minutes, others, for forty-five minutes, depending on the illness. Since I was dealing with acute care only, many of my patients came in once and I never saw them again. I wasn't doing much health maintenance, prevention, or chronic disease management. There's a whole different set of issues that comes up when you're dealing with the long term. I knew it would be much more interesting to be involved with continuing care.

Still, with some of my cases, I did have a chance to make a difference. One afternoon a young man named Scott came in complaining that he was having trouble breathing. I diagnosed him as having asthma and gave him a prescription for some medication. On his way out the door, Scott stopped me and said, "By the way, I wanted to ask you about something else. The other day in the shower, I noticed this thing that feels like a lump on my testicle." I examined him right away. It was very clear to me that he had testicular cancer. By the next morning, he was in surgery with the urologist I'd consulted. Scott did very well with aggressive treatment and radiation therapy. For the next several years, he would stop by and visit me in my office and thank me for saving his life.

That winter, I got a phone call from one of the families I had taken care of during my residency at the hospital's family health center. I delivered their baby while I was there and took care of him as an infant. The parents, Jim and Angela, told me that their son, Alex, who was about six months old, had just died after falling off a couch. They wanted to talk to me about it because they were so grief-stricken. It was one of the times when I realized I really missed that kind of care, where I had ongoing relationships with my patients. I enjoyed getting to know people and their families over time; I also missed working with children and delivering babies.

When you have a history with a family that goes back a number of years like that, and you've been part of major events in their lives, you have a different relationship. Today, in my own practice, I have some families that have been with me now for ten or twelve years—I have delivered their babies, seen them through operations, and helped them cope with death. I've found that knowing people that well helps you put their problems in context.

One of my patients, a working guy in his early forties named Dale, called the office and asked the nurse about high blood pressure symptoms. I knew that Dale rarely spoke up if something was wrong, so I asked him to schedule an appointment with me. When Dale came in, I asked him what was bothering him. He looked at me and said, "Lately, when I'm at work and I run up a flight of stairs, it feels like my collar is too tight, and my head starts pounding around my ears."

"Have you been having headaches?" I asked.

"No," he said. "It just kind of feels like this pressure in my head. It always goes away after about twenty minutes."

If I didn't know Dale so well, I probably wouldn't have taken his complaint as seriously as I did. Even though his physical exam was normal and he didn't have any other symptoms, I went ahead and ordered a CAT scan of his brain. When the results came back, it turned out that he was having increased intracranial pressure from a brain tumor.

It's only after many years of practice that I've come to realize how important it is to know your patients and to listen to them carefully. It makes such a difference in your ability to sort through symptoms. The challenge of primary care is sorting out a problem from its beginning. Health problems are often subtle. It can take weeks or even months to diagnose something. It's an intellectual challenge. More than anything else, it's a tremendous detective game.

It was the intellectual challenge that first attracted me to medicine, but it took me a while to get there. When I was growing up in Buffalo, New York, I used to follow my father, who was a neurologist, while he did his rounds in the hospital on Sundays after church. I watched him as he went from patient to patient. He always held their hands, and it seemed like he spent a long time talking with them. He had a very caring bedside manner. Those early experiences sparked my interest in medicine and made me feel comfortable in a hospital atmosphere.

I always wanted to be a doctor, but I was raised in a pretty conservative Catholic Italian family in which most of the girls did not pursue higher education. It was just not encouraged—if I was interested in health care, it would certainly be nursing, not medicine. So I went to nursing school. I loved being in the hospital and I loved taking care of patients, but I was bored. I took a lot of extra courses, but I still didn't feel challenged. Later, I dropped out and switched to a liberal arts program at the University of Buffalo. It hadn't sunk in to my brain that being a doctor was something I could do. But the fascination was there.

While I was in college, I worked nights as a nurse's aide in the intensive care unit and the emergency room at the local hospital, where I often assisted the doctors with procedures. I can remember saying to the head nurse there, "I'm as smart as these guys, I could do what they do." She always said, "You're right. Why don't you?" But I didn't listen. It was part of my upbringing that being a doctor just wasn't what girls did.

Then I enrolled in a four-year baccalaureate nursing program, thinking the academics might be harder and more challenging. A few days before I was supposed to start, I told my parents that I wanted to pursue a premed major instead. They were shocked. I was the oldest in a family of eight kids, and while they were supportive, they didn't quite know what to make of it.

After I enrolled in medical school, the leaps in personal growth that occurred for me were amazing. I was doing exactly what I wanted. Finally, I felt challenged intellectually.

One reason I dismissed the idea of going into medicine when I was growing up was that people told me it was absolutely impossible to be a doctor and a mother at the same time. I encountered this attitude throughout my medical training. For example, when I got pregnant as a resident, I tried to arrange my schedule so I could be on call more in the beginning and less in the end, as I got closer to my due date, but they wouldn't let me do it. There wasn't much understanding of what it's like to be pregnant. You're still expected to be up for thirty-six hours, running around the hospital.

The first year with the baby, fatigue became the norm. He was ten weeks old when I started at the student clinic, and I was torn up about going to work and being away from him. Luckily, I was able to arrange for my mother-in-law to take care of him in our home during the day. Since I was breast-feeding for the first eleven months, I used a breast pump and left the milk for him while I was away. Breast-feeding my baby made me feel closer to him. That was a way

I could immediately connect with him when I came home. It also helped him sleep better through the night. I also nursed my daughter, Amelia, when she was born five years later.

Today, the biggest challenge for me continues to be arranging child care. In my family practice now, I deliver a lot of babies, so I have to leave in the middle of the night. I have a college student who has agreed to be on call for me. She wears a beeper, so if I get called, she'll come right over and stay with the kids until I get back.

My children have asthma and allergies. When they are sick, it's always difficult to figure out who is going to be able to care for them. If you call in and say you're not going to be in that day, there are twenty patients who need to be rescheduled. It's a very difficult situation, but my kids have grown up with it, and they are very happy, secure, well-adjusted children.

It would probably have been easier for me to work for a health maintenance organization (HMO) from nine to five, but I work around my schedule because I love what I'm doing. Primary care is very challenging. I believe that there is absolutely no reason on earth to think that being a doctor and raising a family aren't compatible. Any profession is going to present challenges in terms of having children. There are so many options, you can do anything you want in medicine and still be a good mother.

Incidentally, when my son, Zachary, needed an operation for a hernia a few years ago, I told him he would be seeing a male surgeon. He looked at me, surprised, and asked, "Mommy, boys can't be doctors, can they?" So there I was, trying to explain to my four-year-old son that boys can be anything they want, just like girls.

Mary Alfano is a family practice physician in Michigan.

12

Office Romance

 S U S A N B R E E N

I was a third-year student at Johns Hopkins when I met my husband, Tom. He was a general surgery resident in the emergency room, where I was doing a one-month elective rotation. I hadn't really talked to him much until we had a tremendous trauma case brought in by helicopter.

The patient was a drug dealer who had just killed a policeman in a raid and who had himself been shot in the chest and leg when he tried to escape. I can recall the windows of the trauma room being plastered with the faces of the deceased officer's colleagues, who likely did not care if the man lived or died. Tom took me through several invasive procedures to stabilize the patient. Blood was everywhere. It certainly wasn't the most romantic of meeting places, but that's how we first got to know each other.

We got married five years later, after I finished my internship in Baltimore, and my ophthalmology residency at Cornell/New York Hospital. We moved to Massachusetts, where Tom had an academic position in orthopedic surgery at the University of Massachusetts Medical Center, and I joined a large multispecialty group practice.

We had an interesting first year in practice because it was also the first year of our marriage. It was the first time we'd been together for an extended period of time in three years, as we used to commute every few weekends between Boston, where Tom was doing a hand-surgery fellowship, and New York, where I did my residency. It was almost harder to adjust to being married and living with someone than to get accustomed to my new practice situation. Even such relatively minor details as who would pay the student loan bills or who would shop for dinner became a study in logistics.

Two-physician couples can be under a great amount of stress. I feared it would potentially jeopardize our chances for a successful marriage. That was something I did not want to risk, so I started out working a little bit less than full-time. In this way, we got many of our errands done during the day, leaving the evenings more free to relax and be together. I feel like I made very good choices. I had enough partners in my practice to be on call once every several weeks. I was home early a couple of afternoons a week and had free time to spend with Tom on most weekends.

Our courtship was one of great understanding. Tom and I used to cook together a lot even though we lived across town from each other during my internship in Baltimore. I can recall coming home after a twenty-four-hour shift at the hospital and collapsing on the couch. I awakened to find that Tom had candles lit on the table and dinner ready. That understanding lasted after we were married and helped us get through a stressful first year. We continued to share cooking responsibilities. Whoever got home first would empty the dishwasher and start dinner. We both had board-certification exams in our specialties later that year, so a good part of our evenings were spent studying.

When I first got to medical school in Baltimore, I had almost vowed not to marry someone who was in medicine. Until my third year, the guys that I dated were all business students or attorneys. I can remember one afternoon when I had plans to meet a lawyer I was seeing for dinner after work. A patient on my team developed a sudden high fever and became quite ill just before we were to sign out to the covering team. The intern and I stayed to look after her, and I had to cancel our date at the last minute. Episodes like that quickly led to the end of that relationship.

So during our first year, if Tom came home two hours late one day, I would understand because it probably happened to me the week before. Or if I had a tough case in the operating room, Tom understood that I couldn't just leave my feelings about it at the office.

Part of choosing a spouse is simply who you happen to meet, no matter what your profession. Most people tend to meet their spouses while in their twenties or early thirties. You're in the hospital so much as a medical student and resident that it naturally becomes a major source of friends and romantic partners. I suppose there's a certain trench mentality to medical training; it creates a bond that lasts a lifetime. After the collegiality of medical school and residency, working on my own in a private practice was a difficult adjustment. It's a very solitary life, and seems especially so after being in a large, amorphous crowd for so many years.

One of the benefits of being in a group practice was that if I had a very tough case, I could ask my colleagues down the hall for advice. I also avoided having to deal with the business headaches such as furnishing an office, buying equipment, and interviewing support staff. I probably made less money than I could have made in solo practice, but I didn't have to worry about the hiring and firing aspect of it.

Ninety-five percent of my work was cataract extraction. The vast majority of my patients were over sixty years old and had glaucoma or cataracts, although I also saw children for other eye diseases. My day usually started at eight or eight-thirty. I spent three and a half days a week seeing patients in the office, and one day a week in the operating room. On a typical day, I would see about thirty-five patients by about four o'clock; most nights, I got home by five or five-thirty. While I was in school, I didn't fully realize how much of the doctor/patient relationship involves teaching. Sometimes I got frustrated with having to explain what glaucoma is ten times a day. I spent one day a week doing mostly outpatient cataract surgery at the hospital.

Ophthalmology is evolving so rapidly that by the end of my first year of practice, I was already converting to an entirely new approach to the removal of cataracts called phacoemulsification. I was fortunate to share operating time with a colleague who was quite adept at this technique, so my conversion to this newer method could be a gradual apprenticeship. As in residency, I first observed many cases. Then, after practicing with the surgical instrumentation at several courses, I began to do more and more on my own.

The transition from residency to practice was most acutely evident to me in the operating room. In residency, a faculty surgeon is always in attendance for surgical cases. As an attending surgeon, suddenly I was the one in charge in the operating room. The overall tone set by the surgeon carries over to the entire staff of nurses, anesthetist, and technicians. It was a new, empowering, yet humbling feeling to be the one ultimately in charge of the entire surgical "performance." I needed to determine every aspect of the case, from the appropriateness of the surgical indications to the exact needles and sutures used. I often wished that I had paid attention to more of those details when I was finishing my residency. Occasionally I found myself on the phone with the head nurse in the O.R. at Cornell, asking her which needles we had used for different cases.

I think if I could somehow repeat this transition, I might have benefited from spending time seeing how the attending surgeons who taught us in residency ran their own practices—from billing to equipment. I think these comparisons and experienced opinions would be invaluable when you have to choose from so many options entering any type of practice.

I truly love what I do. I have a wonderful general ophthalmology practice, and by virtue of being in a larger group practice, I have been able to cut back my schedule even further since the birth of our son, Ryan. I sometimes yearn for the perhaps missed opportunity of further specialization within ophthalmology, but the intensive fellowship period alone may have put too much of a strain on my marriage. In nearly all of the marriages of my female friends in medicine, they have been the ones who have made the most adjustments in their practices and sacrifices in their careers. It takes very careful planning to find or create a practice that can accommodate the tribulations of marriage and motherhood, but combining all these roles can be a great source of joy.

Susan Breen is an ophthalmologist at a clinic in Massachusetts.

13

Uncommon Heroes

Occasionally I run into people who make me stop for a minute and examine my hectic but privileged life. These people make me remember why I chose medicine as a career. They endure so visibly, and with such good cheer, in my memory. Donna is one of those people. She was my patient during my first year doing prenatal and obstetric care for people with problem pregnancies.

Donna was heroic in my eyes. She was five feet, two inches tall, and she weighed about 365 pounds. She could not walk more than a few steps without gasping for breath. Because of the extra weight, Donna had significant medical problems, including diabetes, hypertension, and sleep apnea. Donna was married to a migrant worker. They lived on a poor income in government-subsidized housing.

Her family life was brighter than her physical condition. Her husband, by all accounts, was loving and supportive of Donna and their children. They had difficulties with their children, though. Donna's first child died of sudden infant death syndrome (SIDS), one month after it was born. Another pregnancy ended in stillbirth. Her oldest son, a young teen, was diagnosed with attention deficit disorder and required special schooling. She had a daughter and another son who were healthy, bright, interactive children.

I got to know Donna when she came in for prenatal care during her most recent pregnancy. The county she lived in had limited prenatal care, especially for Medicaid recipients. So Donna would get on a bus at 5:30 A.M. and make a two-hour trip for her appointments with me. She made arrangements beforehand with her sister and a friend to make sure her children got to school those mornings. Donna had to go through all this trouble because no one in her area was willing to give her the medical care she needed during her complicated pregnancy.

Before she came to us, she endured some insulting treatment from other health care providers. One person felt it was so important to know Donna's exact weight, he sent her to the hospital loading dock to be weighed, as if she were freight. Many people told her that she had no business having another child because she had no money and so many health problems. Few people cared how she felt, and few understood that she had no choices once she was pregnant.

But she persisted, with an unshakable positive attitude. Donna appreciated everyone—she saw only the good in those who cared for her, and she brightened up our lives. She delivered a healthy, beautiful daughter. Two weeks later, Donna died of cardiac arrhythmia suddenly and unexpectedly at home. To me, she was a true heroine because of the way she dealt with the obstacles that stood in her way and still managed to get good health care for her child.

I love what I do. But the politics and financial concerns that revolve around medicine as a business can make this line of work unpalatable. It is that side of medicine as a career that occasionally makes me question the road I've traveled so far. My choice of obstetrics is further complicated by family obligations. I sometimes long for a more normal family life with regular hours and nights and weekends at home. The lifestyle of an obstetrician is rarely conducive to this more traditional schedule, for both women and men. Others rarely understand our long and frequently unpredictable hours. Sleep deprivation, although inconstant, is a very real part of my lifestyle. Babies do not decide to come only between the hours of 9:00 A.M. and 5:00 P.M. Even when I am not on call or at the hospital, my concern about patients can take my attention away from family matters.

Would I choose a different career knowing what I do now? Probably not. Nothing, absolutely nothing, compares with the thrill of delivering a wanted, healthy baby. At the same time, nothing compares to the heartbreak of unhealthy mothers having unhealthy babies. A friend once told me I had taken a generally happy field, obstetrics, and turned it into a depressing one by specializing in problem pregnancies. While that viewpoint is certainly valid, I stick by my choice because I have been able to help people at such a critical point in their lives. I feel strongly that if we support mothers who have problem pregnancies during this difficult time, it may make a difference for them.

A great many women I cared for my first year used illicit drugs, such as cocaine or heroin, or alcohol during their pregnancies. Instead of turning our backs on them, we gave them comprehensive care with the hope that we could have a positive influence on their lives and their children's lives. We collected some preliminary data to show that if people get good prenatal care, the chances of low-birthweight babies and preterm delivery are fewer. The data also hold true for women who use cocaine. These factors can have a profound effect on the future well-being of these children.

Two of the women from our special care clinic returned with their healthy babies to say that they stopped using drugs because we treated them like human beings during their prenatal care. Both were cocaine abusers. One of the women, Leticia, was jailed for selling drugs prior to becoming pregnant. She has a little boy who was a terror. We helped her enroll in a class where she could learn some parenting skills while her son was in day care. She is learning to control him better, which is wonderful. At the same time, the classes also helped Leticia boost her self-esteem.

Leticia started coming to the clinic when she was about three and a half months pregnant. We saw her regularly during the months that led up to her delivery. Sometimes we talked about how things were going for her. Other times, she was too high to be coherent. Many of us want to ask these women, "How can you do this to yourself? How can you do this to your baby?" But I don't preach because preaching makes them not want to come anymore, and makes them turn to drugs even more. We talked to her about her life and her kids instead of telling her she was a horrible person. When she came back after her baby was born, Leticia told us that we inspired her to make a change. She said that if we liked her as much as we did even when she was on drugs, we would like her even more when she stopped. Obviously, Leticia was a special case. To assume we could have that effect on most substance abusers would be unrealistic. But it is a step in the right direction.

It is the needy women like Leticia and Donna who gave my job meaning. Patients' needs came in many forms, colors, and styles. I worked with people whose pregnancies were complicated by medical problems, the woes of poverty, substance abuse, or spouse abuse. Others simply experienced the normal aches and pains of being pregnant.

Working with Tina, who happened to be pregnant at the same

time I was, was an experience that helped me empathize with my patients in a very direct way. I first met Tina three years ago, when she was pregnant with her first child. By coincidence, we happened to have the same due date. I was expecting a normal, healthy girl, which I got. Tina was expecting a normal, healthy boy. After we did an ultrasound, I had the unenviable task of explaining that her little boy had severe urinary tract abnormalities and would probably not survive. When this turned out to be true, I cried with Tina and her husband. When her second pregnancy was also anomalous, and the fetus died in utero, I cried for her again. Recently, though, I cried tears of joy with Tina the day she delivered a beautiful, normal, and healthy daughter.

Women were certainly able to have babies long before there were obstetricians. No doubt, they would still be doing so without us. But I believe we can make the experience easier and safer much of the time. The downside of this specialty is that you always feel like you've shortchanged some part of your life because the hours are so demanding. I am lucky. I have a fabulous husband who not only puts up with all this but also is as dedicated to raising my child as I am. Unfortunately, many women do not have this support, making such a career choice difficult. There is nothing in the world like obstetrics. I can't imagine doing anything else.

Jacki Howitt is the perinatologist at Rochester General Hospital and assistant professor of obstetrics at the University of Rochester in Rochester, New York.

14

The Front Lines of Emergency Medicine

 BRENDA MERRITT

I spent my first year as a doctor in the South Bronx, in one of the busiest emergency rooms in the country. Ambulances were constantly pulling up to the doors to unload more patients. There were so many people to take care of, we sometimes ran out of stretchers. I could never conceive of catching up and seeing all the patients—I just had to try to see the sicker ones first.

Some days I could barely find time to sit down and catch my breath. The long hours never bothered me, though. My shift was supposed to be from 8:00 A.M. to 4:00 P.M., but I don't think I ever left that emergency room before six-thirty at night, and I didn't take lunch breaks. I thrived on the hectic pace. It made me feel powerful to be able to do this well and see the results of my work immediately. I left at the end of the day exhausted but incredibly satisfied.

The area I worked in looks like an average inner-city neighborhood. It has burned-out buildings, large tenements, garbage and stray dogs on the street, people strung out on drugs, and families trying to function in the midst of it. I grew up in the Bronx, so I felt comfortable there. I thought I could learn the most at a large city hospital, and it made me feel good to give something back to my community.

Forming close relationships with some of my regular patients added to my first year in the emergency room, but it also forced me to learn a hard lesson: Doctors can't fix everything. Sometimes diseases like AIDS and chronic social problems get in the way, no matter how much training you've had. People in the community were very poor. They often did not have access to preventive health care. Any diseases they had weren't taken care of until they became so sick they had to come into the hospital. There was also a lot of violence in the community. We saw a high volume of trauma cases—gunshot wounds, stabbings, and violence related to drugs. Many of the patients who came to the emergency room were mentally ill. Some were unable to think clearly because they were psychotic. Once in a while, patients who appeared psychotic actually had some other medical problem that affected their thinking.

One night a seventy-year-old man named Ernest came in. He was diabetic and had taken too much insulin. He had no sugar in his blood, which made him extremely violent and confused. I had to get sugar into him or he was going to die. It was hard because he was screaming and throwing punches as I tried to start an intravenous in his arm. I really got hurt. As the sugar level rose in his body, he woke up. Suddenly, he became this sweet older gentleman. In a soft voice, he asked, "Why do you have me in restraints like this?"

"You were acting very agitated and confused a while ago," I explained. "We had to tie you down to get the sugar into your blood or you would have died."

"What is that mark on your face?" he asked.

I told him that I got a couple of bruises when I tried to give him the injection. He was incredulous. "I did that?" he said. "I really beat you up? I'm so sorry!"

After that combative start, Ernest and I forged a friendship as he recovered. The incident helped me to understand psychotic illness better. Certainly, people with psychosis would also like to be able to take a medicine that would allow them to wake up and function normally again. For some of the mentally ill patients I saw, that option simply did not exist.

Since many of the people in the South Bronx don't have health insurance, they relied on our emergency room as their primary health care provider. There was always a crowd of people waiting to be seen. They would often sit there all night, waiting for an average of six hours to be treated for a sore throat or a cut finger because we were so busy taking care of the more serious cases. A lot of heartbreaking cases of poverty, drug abuse, child abuse, and rape came through our doors. But what got to me the most was when there was nothing I could do to help.

When someone came in with a gunshot, I could fix that. I could take out the bullet, and if the person made it, the event was over. It was harder with some of the homeless people we used to see regularly. People who don't have a home are often mentally ill. They spend a lot of time walking. Their legs swell and they frequently develop ulcers because the skin gets so thin. I got to know a homeless man named Kevin who sometimes came in with open, pus-filled ulcers on his legs. He was about fifty and he had schizophrenia. He had a scruffy red beard and layers of torn clothing. He always carried a shopping bag and a walking stick. I would give him a prescription for antibiotics and tell him to keep his feet up while they healed, but I knew he didn't have the money to buy the medicine. And he had no place to go where he could put his feet up. I did what I could for him, but I knew I was just sending him back to the street. A week later, he would show up again with the same problem. It was frustrating. I felt as if I should have been able to tackle that, but the system didn't allow for it. Now the city has better outreach programs to get people into shelters so they can get the medical attention they need. When I first started out in practice, those programs weren't in place yet.

The AIDS epidemic was also just beginning then, and we had no idea what we were dealing with. I had a patient named Roberto who came to the emergency room every time he got really sick. No one knew what was the matter with him. Roberto had a wife and four kids who usually came in with him, and over time, I got to know his family well, which is unusual for an emergency room. Most patients are in and out within a few hours, so you don't form any lasting bonds with them. It's easier to see them once, fix their problem, and never see them again. It was hard for me to stand by and let Roberto's children watch their father die when no one knew what was wrong or what to do for him.

I used to get into heated discussions with the infectious disease doctor about Roberto's condition. I thought Roberto had all the signs and symptoms of atypical tuberculosis, but the other physician was convinced it had something to do with his immune system. We kept arguing back and forth about it. Meanwhile, the patient kept coming back sicker and sicker.

"He clearly has TB," I used to say to the other physician. "I don't understand why you're not starting the TB medicine."

He always answered me the same way. "I don't think he has TB. It's obvious that he has some form of immune suppression," he said. "That's what's going on."

In the end, we were both right. I now know that he had AIDS with atypical TB. Roberto died a few months after I first met him. I can still see his face. It was the typical hollow face of someone dying of AIDS, but I didn't know that at the time. He kept coming back with infections that got progressively worse. I felt helpless.

We didn't take any precautions back then. I didn't know enough about the disease to wear protective gloves or a mask. I was literally so busy in the emergency room that I would take a bite out of a sandwich and put it down on a bloody table while I worked. We never worried about something like eating in blood.

During my first year as an emergency physician, I also formed close relationships with some of the people who suffered from severe asthma. They had such difficulty breathing that they had to be in the emergency room every day of their lives. We had an area called the asthma room that had about thirty people getting treatment all the time. The doctors on staff used to take turns being assigned to the asthma room. At the hospital where I spent my first year, there was an unusually high number of asthma cases. I'm not sure what caused it, but it may have been the poor air quality in the South Bronx. Also, we had a large population of Hispanic patients who may have a genetic predisposition to develop problems with asthma.

There were several women in their sixties who came to the asthma room every day. They brought their bags of knitting and embroidery, prepared to sit all day. Their chairs were arranged in a circle. As I went around the room giving them intravenous medication and listening to their lungs, they would tell me things and ask me about my family. While they waited, the people who were breathing easier chatted with one another about everyday things such as a new hairdo or someone in the community who recently got married. I built up some very intimate relationships with those patients because I saw them every day. They were very special to me.

If one of those people died, which they did on a regular basis, it affected me more than it did the other staff because I knew them so well. The daily routine in the asthma room was often interrupted if someone wasn't doing well. All of a sudden a patient would stop breathing. We would have to rush her out of the room and try to resuscitate her. It was scary for everybody else in the room to watch that. If the person didn't make it, the whole group felt the pain.

I don't think I ever got used to death—it really takes its toll on you. It certainly is very emotionally draining, but it also depends on the case. If a ninety-five-year-old patient is in a vegetative state, dying can sometimes be a relief, an end to a satisfying life. On the other hand, if a two-year-old dies suddenly in an accident, there's nothing more devastating. It affects everyone in the emergency room.

My husband is also a physician. We helped each other cope with the emotional strain and the stress that first year, and we still do, ten years later. When we go home, the first hour is always spent sharing all of the cases of the day. A physician's life is different from that of other people. It's not a job. It's not even a career. It's just a major part of your life that is always there. If you have someone else who understands and can share that with you, it makes your outside life easier.

The people I worked with in the emergency room were also extremely supportive. We worked hard together and we played hard together. It was a family atmosphere. Everybody stayed late, worked hard, and pulled together. No matter what their role was, they were all so dedicated and so willing to give of themselves. In the face of constant obstacles like being understaffed, underpaid, and dealing with bad equipment, people kept their spirit of professionalism. It really made the difference between that hospital being what used to be called a "butcher shop" in the old days, and being one of the finest emergency rooms in the country, despite the horrible conditions.

My first year in the emergency room was physically grueling and emotionally exhausting. But the constant challenge, the diversity of the field, and the strong friendships I developed kept me coming back. My job exposed me to parts of human nature that people in other careers rarely see—extreme poverty, humor, violence, insanity, and courage—but most of all, the chance to save a life.

Brenda Merritt is director of emergency services at a hospital in New York City.

15

The Doctor Hotel

 N. Patrick Hennessey

I began my private dermatology practice in a place I used to call the doctor hotel. It was a four-story building in a good location in Manhattan where I rented office space by the hour. Therapists used the space as did doctors in other specialties. I used to go there in the evenings, after my day job with a prepaid health plan. In the beginning, I had no employees. I had to be the receptionist and office manager in addition to taking care of patients.

Most of the first year of my small private practice, I carried all of my patient files in my briefcase. I had a small cabinet where I could store my things in between visits to the doctor hotel. I didn't have an autoclave or sterilizer for the instruments I used, so I used to dip them in sterilizing solution. At the end of each session, I would pack them in sterile bags and take them with me in my briefcase. The next morning, I ran them through the sterilizer at the prepaid health plan and took them back to the office for the next round of procedures.

The first year of my practice at the doctor hotel was filled with all kinds of revelations about how to run a business. I was responsible for ordering my own supplies, from gauze to toilet paper. A few times, I found myself reaching for some gauze in the middle of a procedure, only to discover that I had used the last package and had forgotten to order more. During my training, I thought things would be easier when I started practicing on my own, but actually my work was just beginning. I was continuing my education as a medical businessman.

Many of my experiences my first year were very amusing. I remember one patient, a stockbroker, who needed a wart removed from her foot. She seemed fine, but she didn't tell me that earlier that day, some friends gave her a handful of drugs so she wouldn't be nervous for the operation. In the middle of the procedure, this very composed stockbroker started sliding all over the table like she was drunk. She moaned and cursed and carried on. I tried to talk her through it and keep her occupied while I worked on her foot. This wart had been there a long time, and a major vessel had worked its way closer to the surface than usual. As she moved around, I managed to slice right into it. Blood was coming out everywhere and splattering the wall of the doctor hotel. At that point, I asked myself, "Why are you doing this? Why did you ever want to do this?" I finally managed to stop the bleeding. By the time the procedure was done, she was drifting off to sleep. She didn't even remember what happened.

Although I laugh at stories like that now, my first year was frustrating and depressing at times. A lot of my friends outside of medicine had already been working for ten years. They were talking about taking expensive vacations and buying homes as I struggled to pay the rent for one more session of patient hours at the doctor hotel. My financial picture was limited by the fact that I chose to start a solo practice in New York City, where the market is extremely competitive for physicians, especially in specialties like dermatology.

I decided to set up my practice in this urban setting because of my sexual orientation toward other men. When my residency was over I was faced with two choices. I could stay in an urban area with a large population of lesbian and gay people to interact with socially and professionally, or I could move to a suburban or rural area of the country where I would have to remain in the closet. I decided earlier in my residency that I wasn't comfortable with having a double life, so the significant decision in terms of where to practice was already made. There was no way I would have stayed anywhere other than a major urban area.

I made the decision to go to medical school twenty years ago, knowing that if I were ever discovered as a gay person, the information could, by law, preclude my getting my license to practice. I stayed in the closet through medical school. Once I graduated, finished my internship, and earned a medical license, I no longer felt that my sexuality threatened my career in medicine. Around the same time, I began to realize that I was living a double life. I didn't like having friends I couldn't introduce to other friends. So, I decided to leave the Midwest and finish my residency in internal medicine at Harvard. When I moved to Boston, I was still questioning whether there were any other gay people in medicine. Fortunately, I did meet people like me there. I went on to do my dermatology training in New York, where I began to feel comfortable about being openly gay.

Although I would not have predicted it, an early experience during my training influenced the path my career would later follow. During the last six months of my residency, we saw the first three cases of Kaposi's sarcoma in New York. I remember talking with the chief resident about how there must be some connection between these three patients. I thought it had to be more than just a freak occurrence that three people would have such an unusual malignancy at the same time. It struck me that these were not the typical people who got Kaposi's sarcoma. The disease usually shows up in older men of southern European or Mediterranean extraction and develops slowly over a period of years. Yet, here we had three patients who were all young men under thirty-five and they all had an aggressive form of the disease.

The chief resident and I did some research, trying to find some correlation. I thought that the two patients I had seen were probably gay. We checked the third patient's medical charts to see if we could turn up any evidence that he might also be gay. The record showed that he was a young, single male who had never been married. Each of these patients had a fair amount of sexually transmitted disease, and they all had hepatitis. We tried to link something about being gay, sexually transmitted diseases, and hepatitis, but there was no clear common denominator yet. When I finished my residency and went into private practice, I set aside that academic work for the time being.

The introduction of HIV into society at large and into the delivery of health care paralleled the end of my residency training and the beginning of when I went into practice on my own. I entered practice with full intentions of pursuing a profession as a general dermatologist. In fact, fourteen years later, I have a practice that is part dermatology and part primary care for AIDS patients.

Toward the end of my first year, I got a note from the colleague I studied the three cases of Kaposi's sarcoma with during my residency. He sent me some newspaper clippings about how patients in California were starting to come down with pneumonia and opportunistic infections. In late 1981, we both began to see how these cases were all interrelated. The AIDS epidemic started to evolve.

I didn't have a sense of the significance of what this was going to mean for medicine, society, and for me as an individual during the first six months of my practice. But certainly by the time I finished the second six months, I began to suspect that something was very wrong. I was seeing too many otherwise healthy young men getting too much skin disease. I saw fungal infections that took much longer to treat than normal. These skin diseases were similar to those of a diabetic patient or someone who was taking immunosuppressant drugs for cancer treatment. These early AIDS cases set the stage for my practice to become more focused on the HIV-related aspects of dermatology. The very first patient I treated in my office for Kaposi's sarcoma came to me after hearing from two other dermatologists that his lesions were nothing to worry about. A friend encouraged him to see me for another opinion. We took a biopsy and found Kaposi's sarcoma.

Clearly, by the end of the first year, you evolve into what characterizes you in your practice. You find your niche in your professional life.

N. Patrick Hennessey is a dermatologist and primary care physician in New York City.

16

The Privilege of Listening

 DAVID PRESTON

The first day I came into my new office, my two internal medicine partners handed me a full schedule of twenty patients to see by five o'clock. Every half hour a new patient came in with a complicated medical history, a long list of ailments, and a unique set of personality traits that I had to sort out in the course of a few minutes. I didn't have time to sit down and think, I just had to do it.

I had just moved to Maine after finishing my internal medicine residency in Boston. In a hospital setting, I was used to seeing patients while surrounded by a team of interns, residents, medical students, and attending physicians. Yet here I was, mostly on my own, in a small factory town on the Kennebec River. Without the security of my old academic setting, I felt as if I was just going by the seat of my pants half the time, not knowing if what I did was right. But a couple of early successes showed me that I could trust my instincts. As the year progressed, I learned that truly listening to patients takes more energy than I expected, but if you're willing to do it, they will reveal everything you need to know to make them healthier. I was surprised that once I earned people's respect as their primary care physician, I could persuade them to prevent future health problems by scheduling a mammogram or giving up cigarettes.

About two months into my first year of practice, the emergency room called from the local hospital to say they were sending me a sixty-five-year-old woman named Helen. When Helen got to my office, she told me another doctor had treated her for sinusitis, but it didn't seem to be working.

"The pills he gave me don't get rid of these headaches I've been having," she said. "I just feel terrible. I ache all over and I can hardly get up in the morning."

I listened carefully to her complaints. One of the diseases that came to mind was temporal arteritis, which is an inflammation of the blood vessels in the head. People who have it can lose their sight suddenly and irreversibly in one or both eyes unless it's diagnosed in time. The first test I ordered, a sedimentation rate, came back very high, so the next day I had a biopsy done on her temporal artery. It was positive, so I started her on an anti-inflammatory medication called prednisone. She came back the next week.

"It's like a miracle!" she said. "I took one pill and I felt better."

When my daughter, Beth, was born the next year, Helen knitted an afghan for my family. I felt proud that I was able to prevent her from losing her vision, and she was so appreciative.

The full spectrum of the community came through my office. We had patients who hadn't had a bath in two weeks and executives with six-figure salaries. Some people worked at a nearby paper mill, others were farmers or college professors.

One of my patients, eighty-year-old Sister Marie, was a French-Canadian nun. She was a stout, white-haired lady with sparkling eyes who first came to my office for a routine physical exam because she hadn't had one in years. She said she was feeling tired and appeared pale and anemic. I asked her all my usual questions including those about abdominal pain and bowel movements.

"I'm going to do a complete, head-to-toe physical exam today," I said.

"Yes, doctor," she said.

"I'm also going to have to check the rectum to make sure everything is okay," I added.

I think she was embarrassed, but I went ahead and did it. There was a trace of blood in her stool, so I persuaded her to have a colonoscopy. Sure enough, she did have a colon cancer, which was localized to the bowel. The cancer was removed by a surgeon, and she was cured. If I hadn't done a rectal exam, she might have died of colon cancer, so Sister Marie was extremely grateful to me. Like Helen, she expressed her gratitude with presents. Every two months or so, she comes in with these wonderful paintings of boats and woodland mountain scenes, which I hang in my office waiting room.

Not all my patients were so receptive to my efforts to improve their health. Hank, for example, was a tougher nut to crack. He was thirty-nine years old, but he looked sixty-five. He was disheveled and not very well washed. He had thin, wispy hair, a craggy face, and nicotine-stained hands. Hank had just gotten out of prison, where he had been for a year or so, serving a term for arson. He said he had a drinking problem, which got him into trouble. This had not been his first time in prison, I gathered from talking with him. After just a few minutes of conversation, he decided he was on a first-name basis with me.

"Dave, I'm having these god-awful pains across my chest. I feel like I'm having a heart attack. I think I'm gonna die," he said. "I told the warden, but he don't give a damn. You could rot in that jail and nobody would notice."

I scheduled a stress test for Hank the next week to find out if he had heart disease, but he showed up at my office again two days later with more severe chest pains. He was having a small heart attack, so I admitted him to the hospital right away. After he recovered, we decided to send him over to a larger hospital in Portland, where he eventually underwent a triple bypass.

Hank didn't have any health insurance. He was a heavy smoker and an alcoholic, a model of self-abuse. He was not a very solid citizen, but he needed treatment for his heart disease, so the hospital picked up the tab. After the operation, I scheduled a follow-up visit with Hank. Undergoing massive open-heart surgery is a very sobering experience for most people, so I thought he might be ready to make some lifestyle changes.

"Hank, you're killing yourself with cigarettes," I said. "Smoking is one of the leading causes of heart disease. Every cigarette you smoke is blocking up your arteries," I said.

"Yeah, Dave, I know," he said. "I'm going to stop this time. I really am. I wouldn't lie to you."

I also set up several appointments for him with a substance abuse counselor and referred him to Alcoholics Anonymous. He stopped drinking every now and then, but not for long. As hard as I tried, I couldn't get Hank to kick his substance abuse habits. Sometimes he would even call me in the middle of the night asking for drugs.

"Dave," he said. "I need some of those Percocets. You gotta help me, Dave. My chest is killing me."

I don't prescribe narcotics like that over the phone, so I usually just told him to take some aspirin. He's still my patient, three years later, and I've started treating his girlfriend, too. They usually come in together, cursing the system or somebody who did them wrong. They're always involved in some custody battle or being evicted. Since I'm the only one who listens to them, they come back to me.

I spent a lot of time listening to patients talk about their grandchildren or about how bad they felt. Listening to people takes a lot of energy. One thing I wasn't expecting was the number of people who came in with psychiatric or emotional problems. There's a real stigma about going to see a psychologist or a psychiatrist; it's a lot more acceptable for many people to go to a medical doctor than a "head doctor." Plus, people put a lot of trust in their primary care doctors and want to feel that their doctors care about them.

I also didn't realize how tired I would be in the evening after working all day. During a typical day my first year, I got to work at about 8:00 A.M. and started to do my rounds with patients who were hospitalized. In the afternoon, I would see patients with less-serious medical problems, like back pain, diabetes, and sore throats. My last patient would usually leave by five o'clock; I'd do my paperwork until six-thirty and then go home. I thought I would have more time to spend with my family, taking advantage of our beautiful location near the mountains and ocean. My wife ended up doing almost all of the housework, which made me feel guilty, and I had to work a lot of holidays, nights, and weekends. There's a big conflict between trying to see enough patients to earn a good living, leaving enough time for each patient, and trying to have a humane pace in your work and your life.

Primary care doctors are at the bottom of the pay scale compared with the procedure-oriented medical or surgical subspecialists. I was disappointed to discover that they also aren't as well respected in the profession, although I think that is gradually changing. If you are interested in primary care now, you are in great demand. Hospitals want primary care physicians, and they are willing to give them financial incentives, such as salary guarantees or loan payback arrangements, to have them in the community.

I found primary care to be the most challenging because you have to know a lot more about a wide range of topics. Your knowledge is broad but not very deep in any one area. Instead of doing twenty cataract surgeries every day, I saw patients who were coming in with something different all the time. By continually seeing people as their personal physician, you can have an impact on their overall health. When you get to know them, it helps you influence them more. Your advice carries weight because they know you're going to ask them about it the next time they come in. It takes a special type of person to be patient with people and do preventive medicine. If you can get them to quit smoking, you've done something far more important than doing a coronary bypass twenty years later, and certainly more cost-effective.

There are very few professions that allow you to maintain your interest over the years, and internal medicine is one of them. You get to be Sherlock Holmes. You get to apply your intelligence and your knowledge of science, and see immediate results. Every patient has something new to offer you. It may not be a rare disease, it may be an afghan they knitted for your baby or sharing their concern about an alcoholic husband. Being able to sit down with them and listen to their problems is a privilege.

David Preston is a general internist in Maine.

17

Cross-Cultural Medicine

 D A V I D   S I M E N S O N

Outside my office window, a man with a cart sold *paletas*, the Mexican version of Popsicles. Nearby, some Laotian children played underneath a shady mulberry tree to escape the summer heat. Across the street, I could see an irrigation canal running beside a field where many of my patients earned their living as seasonal farm workers. The sounds coming through my window—people speaking Spanish and Laotian dialects—became familiar to me as my first year as a family practice physician unfolded. Language was sometimes an impenetrable barrier, but it also enriched my experience.

I moved to California to fulfill my obligation to the National Health Service Corps, which gave me a full scholarship for medical school. When I accepted my assignment at a nonprofit community health center, I did not realize how much the area it was in truly was a melting pot. Two-thirds of my patients were migrant workers and their families. They labored in the fields, orchards, dairies, and canneries of the fertile San Joaquin Valley. In addition to Mexican-American farm workers, I also saw a large number of patients who were Laotian immigrants. In this area, there are actually three different ethnic groups who have emigrated from Laos: the lowland Lao, and two hill tribes, the Hmong and Mien. Members of each group have their own language, history, and dress.

Even with a Hmong translator in our clinic, I would sometimes have great difficulty communicating with my patients. One day, an elderly Mien woman who did not speak Lao or Hmong came in with her daughter, complaining of indigestion. The interview went something like this: "Does she have a burning stomach pain?" I asked. My assistant translated into Lao for the daughter, who did not speak English. She and my translator talked for a while until she understood the question. The young woman and her mother talked back and forth in Mien. The daughter gave an answer in Lao to my assistant, who then told me, "It hurts at night." If I had been concentrating, I would be able to remember the original question I asked. And with luck, the answer would relate to the question.

Cultural differences between my patients and me had an important effect on my practice of medicine. I faced many questions that were not included in my medical training: What are the typical occupational health problems of migrant or seasonal farm workers? How do culture and living environment affect a disease process and its treatment? And why is it that, even with a translator, I sometimes still could not communicate effectively with my patients?

It was not just a matter of a different language. My patients thought differently in the way they viewed the world and even their illnesses. I learned the difference between a disease and an illness. A disease is a medical condition with a cause, a specific set of symptoms, a typical progression, and a treatment. An illness is a person's subjective experience and is modified by culture, social class, and personal experience.

My patients asked me about conditions I had never heard of, such as *empacho* and *caida de mollera*. These are culture-bound syndromes, folk-defined illnesses that exist within the context of a particular culture. However, when examined by someone trained in Western medicine, there is no correlation with modern medical definitions or known diagnoses. *Empacho* is a perceived blockage of the intestines, and *caida de mollera* is a sunken anterior fontanelle, or soft spot, in an infant's head. Their folk-health beliefs explain causes for these conditions, and give nonmedical treatments.

A mother brought in her young son complaining of abdominal pain. I gave him my typical greeting for children, "*Hola*, Miguel, gimme five!" We slapped palms, and he gave a big smile. I try to make children feel comfortable. I ask them about their pets, their bikes, or their teachers; I like them to think that I am a friendly man from across the street rather than a scary doctor with a big needle.

After talking to Miguel for a little while, I spoke with his mother about his stomach pain. I was trying my best to understand his symptoms. My Spanish was not very good during my first year.

"He doesn't want to eat, and his belly swells up," the mother said. She looked worried. "He has pain in his stomach." Her happy little son sat on the exam table without any evidence of distress.

"Does he have any vomiting?" I asked. "Any diarrhea or fever?"

"No, but sometimes he's constipated."

I examined Miguel but could find nothing wrong. His abdomen was soft and not tender.

"Do you think he might have *empacho*?" I asked. The mother looked relieved to have me voice her concern.

"Well, yes, he might," she said.

"I don't think he has *empacho*," I said. "He might be a little constipated." I suggested that he drink more liquids and eat fresh fruit and vegetables and whole wheat bread. Miguel's mother accepted this treatment plan without my having to compromise her cultural beliefs.

Initially, talking to parents about these illnesses was confusing. Then I realized that I did not have to categorize them in the same terms of physiology and pathology used for other diseases. What I did have to understand was the parents' concern, and I had to find out what they believed to be the cause of the condition. Then I looked for a medical illness that might be part of the problem, something I could treat with Western medicines or therapies. If I found no physical problem, I could still reassure the parents that I did not think their child had *empacho* or *caida de mollera*.

I learned that it is better to confirm the patient's concern, and to be reassuring, rather than to attack beliefs about an illness. For cross-cultural patients, the process of accepting a new culture and a new style of medical treatment is gradual. They can add new ideas or beliefs to their cultural context without abandoning their own cultural heritage. Many of my patients continue to have culturally based fears of surgery or of pelvic examinations years after I have tried to explain the reason for them.

It takes more than just patience for me to deal with these cross-cultural misunderstandings. I have learned three steps to effective cross-cultural medicine. The first is respect for the patients' cultural values, their way of dress, and their concerns. What is the ideal family size? What is a normal breakfast? Should children wear shoes, socks, or underwear? The American way is not the only way, and I can tell you that I often saw different answers to each of these questions in my first year in practice. I had to believe that each person's cultural context offered answers just as valid as mine.

Once a Laotian shaman came to me for stomach pain. He would often perform rituals to relieve people of various ailments. I asked him, without any sarcasm, if he had tried to cure his own illness, and why he had come to me. He said through the translator that his illness was not a Buddhist type of problem. He saw no inconsistency on his part in coming to a Western doctor, so neither did I.

The second step is understanding. What do my Mexican patients eat for breakfast? Some eat scrambled eggs with cactus (delicious), and others eat corn flakes. What caused that perfectly circular ecchymosis (or hickey) on a Laotian woman's forehead? Suction is applied under a small cup, as a treatment for headache. What does Shuhab, the name of a Sudanese-American infant, mean? It means "falling star." As I increased my understanding of each patient's way of life, I was better able to help improve his or her health. But understanding can only begin on the foundation of respect. Why learn how others deal with the problems of life if you have no respect for their solutions?

The third step is true caring—for the patient and his or her health. During medical school, my closest relationship was with my textbooks. During residency I was closest to the other residents with whom I worked each day. As I started medical practice, I began to develop stronger relationships with my patients. I better understood my patients—their different languages, dress, foods, and beliefs—and I saw many qualities to admire. People who were at first strange and incomprehensible became individuals. I tell my patients that they are in charge of their own health and their health problems. My job is not to dictate their behavior but to give them advice on how they can improve and maintain their health. When

I found myself arguing with a patient, or when communication was closed off because I had offended him or her, it was usually because I had neglected respect or understanding.

In a community as ethnically diverse as this one, some of the people who came from other countries brought unusual diseases with them. I treated many problems during my first year of practice that I never thought I would see when I was a medical student. After seeing patients with these unusual diseases, I would often sit down and read about the problem before going on to see the next patient. This, and inefficiency in charting, made for some long days in the first few months.

One afternoon, a tall, thin man came in with his daughter, who was about ten years old. She had long, wavy black hair. She sat on the exam table while he sat in a chair in the corner of the exam room. He was afraid that he and his daughter had been poisoned by pesticides. He told me what had happened a week earlier.

"Last week they were spraying in the fields near our house. It was dark, and this fog was out in the street. It came in through the window that was cracked open. Me and my daughter started to choke."

"What did you feel like?" I asked.

"Well, Missy was choking, and her stomach hurt."

"Was she sick to her stomach?"

"Yes," he said. "She threw up twice."

"Was she sweating a lot?" I asked.

He said she was. "A while later, a police car came by with its lights flashing. They told us all that we had to leave our homes right away. When I went back to the house the next day, you could still smell it."

I learned that the fields had been sprayed with guthion, an organophosphate pesticide. Due to the wind and the weather, the poison had drifted into their homes. He had heard that some other people had been ill due to the pesticide exposure, and he wanted to see if he and his daughter were all right.

Because I had taken a toxicology course in college, I recognized these symptoms as organophosphate poisoning. But that subject was so impersonal back then, it was just more chemical reactions and enzymes to memorize. I never expected to see anyone who had been poisoned. I reported the cases to the Environmental Health Department, which already knew of the incident. By that time, the father was well again, and Missy's symptoms were resolving. I drew blood tests on them both for the effects of organophosphates.

The Laotian and Mexican immigrants were hosts for a variety of parasites. Tulane Medical School, which I attended, is well known for its School of Tropical Medicine. We spent more time on parasitology than most other medical schools did. There were dozens of bizarre life cycles to memorize. Each has different hosts, larval forms, and paths through the human body as it matures and reproduces. Here was another area that I thought would never be useful in real practice. It seemed like these organisms did not exist outside of the textbook and microscope slides.

I kept a growing list of all the parasites I saw as time went on: flukes, tapeworms, hookworms, and amoebas. The variety of parasites was so impressive that I created a bulletin called "Parasitology Can Be Fun." It was a grimly humorous review of symptoms, diagnosis, and treatment of some strange parasite that had caught my attention. I posted it in our clinic and sent a copy to the head of the public health department lab, who I called often to ask about unusual parasite lab results.

I spent hours looking at slides while in medical school studying tropical medicine. If anyone had told me, while I was studying blood smears infected with *Plasmodium malariae*, that I would actually treat a case of malaria in practice, I wouldn't have believed it.

Yet I did treat a case of malaria in a farm worker who contracted the infection in Mexico. While attending medical school, I toured the leprosarium in Carville, Louisiana. If someone had told me that I would later treat Hansen's disease (leprosy), I would have been equally skeptical. I have since performed several skin biopsies to diagnose Hansen's disease. It is the unexpected and unusual case that adds interest to the routine of treating common conditions.

My first year of medical practice was a turning point in many ways. Learning to adjust to cultural differences was part of the process. As a medical student and resident I admired and was awed by the authority and responsibility assigned to a physician. As I started in practice, it felt strange to take that role myself. I'll never forget the feeling when I treated my first case of bacterial meningitis. There was no senior resident watching over my shoulder when I performed the lumbar puncture to get a specimen of spinal fluid. No attending faculty would come by each day to talk about the choice of antibiotics or the patient's progress. This role as detective, decision maker, and dispenser of treatments is a source of both gratification and insecurity.

During my medical training, the breadth and depth of medical knowledge would sometimes overwhelm me. We were all striving to build a fully functional base of medical knowledge. As I started practice, it was intensely painful to face a situation I did not know how to handle. There was the fear that others would think I was incompetent. There was also the fear that something terrible would happen to the patient because I did not order the best treatment or test. This is another subject never taught in medical school.

I no longer expect to know everything. I have learned where to turn for help, what texts or journals to read, and what consultants can give useful advice. I found out how rewarding it is to have patients give you their trust. I have also learned to accept and respect their culture and their concerns. It is enriching to understand the beauty and variety of other ways of life. Above all, I have learned to meet patients on their own terms.

David Simenson is a family physician at a nonprofit community health center in California.

18

Medicine Man

 ALLEN DOBBS

As my family and I drove from San Diego to Pine Ridge, South Dakota, I reviewed all the things people told me about the reservation and the Oglala Lakota people who lived there. Pine Ridge had the worst reputation at the Indian Health Service. It is difficult to pinpoint the origin of this reputation, but it may have been the history of the massacre at Wounded Knee or the more recent events surrounding the birth of the American Indian movement. In any case, there were rumors of poor relations with whites, and that included health care providers. I heard that several physicians were shot at in the past and that outsiders weren't particularly welcome. I had my own preconceived notions about the place much as I tried to have an open, wait-and-see attitude. Later, I discovered it was nothing like what I'd heard.

About 20,000 people live on the 6,000-square-mile reservation, which covers three counties. The northern part of the reservation includes Badlands National Park. We drove through the Black Hills on the western border on the way to the thirty-five-bed institution where I was to work in family practice. The hospital is situated on the southern border, where the old Indian agency was when the reservation was first formed. All the doctors and nurses work for the Indian Health Service, which is a branch of the U.S. Public Health Service. On the way in, it struck me how immense the land was. The terrain was varied. We passed pine-covered ridges and rolling prairies that always seemed to change colors subtly. There's a lot of wildlife out here—golden eagles, antelope, and deer. At night, you can drive for two hours without seeing a man-made light. It's just you and the stars. It's a humbling experience to be out on the prairie and see how small you are in relation to the rest of the universe. This is the sort of place that forces you to look closer and to look expansively at the same time. It's full of paradoxes.

I came to this hospital after years of medical training, but I encountered a few things medical school had not prepared me for. My first day on the job was not easy. Morale at the hospital was very low. The Indian Health Service had just fired the acting hospital administrator, who was well liked by the staff. Without stopping to introduce themselves, the other physicians started talking about a walk-out. Luckily, it didn't materialize. Most were just suffering from the symptoms of being overworked. Despite all the unrest, I found that just getting in and seeing patients was enjoyable. My job was varied; I took care of people in the emergency room, delivered babies, assisted in the operating room, and ran a tuberculosis clinic. One of the first things I did was resuscitate a newborn baby I had delivered. I had to use everything I was trained to do to stabilize the baby, and he did well.

The overall physical health of people on the reservation is pretty poor. Their life expectancy is much shorter than that of the average American, and they have lots of problems with diabetes, heart disease, cancer, accidents, and alcoholism. It's sad, but it's something I was trained to address as a physician. When I first got there, I was on call every third night and two out of three weekends. I would basically work thirty-six hours straight every third day because I had to be at the clinic the morning after I had been on call all night. It was hard work, but I was doing a lot of good medicine. People really need doctors, and their contributions can make a significant impact.

In medical school we were taught to pay attention to body language when taking medical histories and make lots of eye contact with the patients. But in Lakota culture, if you look someone in the eye for a long time, it's an aggressive behavior that is considered an insult. No one told me about that. I found that out the hard way, and it made taking medical histories very difficult. I first noticed it when I was taking care of patients in the emergency room. When I tried to take a history, the people wouldn't look me in the eyes. I would try to bend down to catch their view, and sometimes I was met with an angry look that made me realize I was stepping on some tender ground or pushing a little too hard. Now, when I take a history, I will look them in the eye briefly and then continue to explain my point looking slightly away.

This was something I could never have learned in medical school. Medical school simply can't teach you everything you need to know. It can only prepare you to learn more in the future. You just have to gear yourself to learn on a constant basis and be receptive to different ideas about people and health care.

One night, an eighteen-year-old man came to the emergency room after being bitten by a rattlesnake. When it first happened, he went to see a medicine man on the reservation. Shortly afterward, he participated in a sundance ceremony, where he fasted for four days. The culmination of this four-day vision quest is a ceremony where people pierce the skin on their chest with a piece of bone and tie a leather thong to it. The other end of the leather thong is attached to the top of a tall sundance structure. Those who take part in the ceremony lean back until the thong draws tight and eventually pops off, breaking the skin. This eighteen-year-old did pretty well, but after fasting for four days, he got sick again and had to come in to the hospital. He had recurring symptoms of leg cramps, nausea, and tremors. He made it clear that he did not like to see physicians.

Two types of medicine men live on the reservation. One is an herbalist who specializes in poultices and medicinal treatments; another looks at the wholeness of the individual and addresses spiritual as well as health needs. For instance, some couples see a medicine man when they have marital problems. Some exchange vows again with him once a year and try to right the wrongs of the previous year. I met some of the medicine men and have often sent the residents who train at the hospital out to talk with them. But I don't think they would be very open to talking about their specific ceremonies and treatments. It's an extreme privilege to be invited to one of those. They don't allow any cameras, and sometimes they don't allow any whites. I have been invited to some of the big traditional ceremonies, like the sundance, and a purification ceremony called a sweat. I also join them to play basketball, which is very big on the reservation.

When people come to work on Indian reservations, they have idealistic perceptions about Native American culture. People come out here expecting *Dances with Wolves* and are disappointed when they see a successful capitalist Native American businessman or, in contrast, a lot of poverty. In fact, Pine Ridge reservation is a very heterogeneous society (different personalities and beliefs), but there's a common thread people share—their history and culture. One of the three counties in the reservation—Shannon County—is the poorest county in the nation, but it has a rich cultural history. The community doesn't have much materialism. When people have a celebration, or a powwow, they'll give away some of their possessions. Giving is emphasized over receiving. It's a pretty common custom, for example, to give somebody a star quilt in appreciation of something. That tradition has been around since at least the turn of the century.

One of the most highly valued character traits of the Lakota people is the ability to really listen without interrupting. As physicians, we're trained to take a medical history, but we're not always trained to be good listeners. This takes time and practice and probably needs more emphasis in medical school. There's always pressure to do more and see more patients. Most of the employees at the hospital are from the Lakota tribe. By getting to know them, I have picked up on their ability to listen.

My interest in Native American culture started when I was growing up in Texas. As an adolescent, I suddenly latched on to the fact that the world was a much bigger place than my local high school. This realization fascinated me. I made several trips through Pueblo Indian country near my grandfather's cabin in New Mexico, which solidified my interest. I grew up in the 1960s when there was a lot of dissatisfaction with modern American culture and a real interest in other cultures. I knew I wanted to go to medical school when I went to college, but all the elective courses I took were related to anthropology and writing.

Both my parents were physicians, and when I was younger, I thought that was the last thing I wanted to do. It just looked like too much work and it didn't seem like fun. Later, I joined the navy. I was a hospital corpsman for three years, but I got tired of being just an employee when I saw what the physicians were doing on a day-to-day basis. They had a lot of self-direction and were helping people. I began to see the profession in a more positive light, so I decided to go back to school. If I could hack it the first year, I would pursue it. I became a career public health service officer at the federal medical school in Maryland.

But it wasn't until I reached the reservation that I was able to fuse my interest in Native American culture and my skill as a doctor. Perhaps this helped me see that different cultures view medicine differently. Their belief systems are different, but many tribes share beliefs about health. Technology-driven modern medicine lacks a connection between spirit, mind, and health. Native American cultures have a much more holistic approach. Modern medicine is just now latching on to the fact that mind, spirit, and body are connected, as three parts of one whole.

My fascination with the way these elements interact prevented me from experiencing burnout, like many physicians who came before me. They were just there to do their two years to pay back government scholarships. After two years, I decided I was here to stay. I found out you can't make so many assumptions about people. And I learned to be a better listener. The most rewarding thing is being able to appreciate individuals within their culture and to understand their ways.

Allen Dobbs is a family practice physician and clinical director in South Dakota.

Index